A PRACTICAL GUIDE
TO THERAPEUTIC
PLASMA EXCHANGE

A PRACTICAL GUIDE TO THERAPEUTIC PLASMA EXCHANGE

Andre A. Kaplan, MD, FACP

Professor of Medicine
University of Connecticut Health Center;
Director, Dialysis Program
John Dempsey Hospital
Farmington, Connecticut

b

**Blackwell
Science**

©1999 by Andre A. Kaplan

Blackwell Science, Inc.
Editorial Offices:
Commerce Place, 350 Main Street, Malden,
  Massachusetts 02148, USA
Osney Mead, Oxford OX2 0EL, England
25 John Street, London WC1N 2BL, England
23 Ainslie Place, Edinburgh EH3 6AJ, Scotland
54 University Street, Carlton, Victoria 3053,
  Australia
Other Editorial Offices:
Blackwell Wissenschafts-Verlag GmbH,
  Kurfürstendamm 57, 10707 Berlin, Germany
Blackwell Science KK, MG Kodenmacho
  Building, 7-10 Kodenmacho Nihombashi,
  Chuo-ku, Tokyo 104, Japan

Distributors:

USA
Blackwell Science, Inc.
Commerce Place
350 Main Street
Malden, Massachusetts 02148
(Telephone orders: 800-215-1000 or 781-388-
  8250; fax orders: 781-388-8270)

Canada
Login Brothers Book Company
324 Saulteaux Crescent
Winnipeg, Manitoba, R3J 3T2
(Telephone orders: 204-224-4068)

Australia
Blackwell Science Pty, Ltd.
54 University Street
Carlton, Victoria 3053
(Telephone orders: 03-9347-0300;
  fax orders: 03-9349-3016)

Outside North America and Australia
Blackwell Science, Ltd.
c/o Marston Book Services, Ltd.
P.O. Box 269
Abingdon
Oxon OX14 4YN
England
(Telephone orders: 44-01235-465500;
  fax orders: 44-01235-465555)

Acquisitions: James Krosschell
Production: Irene Herlihy
Manufacturing: Lisa Flanagan
Typeset by Best-set Typesetter Ltd., Hong Kong
Printed and bound by Braun-Brumfield

Printed in the United States of America
99 00 01 02 5 4 3 2 1

The Blackwell Science logo is a trade mark of
Blackwell Science Ltd., registered at the United
Kingdom Trade Marks Registry

Library of Congress Cataloging-in-Publication
Data

Kaplan, Andre A.
  A practical guide to therapeutic plasma
  exchange / Andre A. Kaplan.
    p. cm.
  Includes bibliographical references and index.
  ISBN 0-632-04395-4 (alk. paper)
  1. Plasma exchange (Therapeutics)—
  Handbooks, manuals, etc.
  I. Title.
  [DNLM: 1. Plasma Exchange—methods
  handbooks. 2. Therapeutics—methods
  handbooks. WH 39 K17p 1999]
  RM175.K37 1999
  615′.39—DC21
  DNLM/DLC
  for Library of Congress   98-33622
                                              CIP

This book is dedicated to my mother's love of learning and my father's love of life

Contents

List of Tables   xiii
List of Figures   xvi
Preface   xviii

PART I: Operating Characteristics

CHAPTER 1
Introduction and Rationale   3

CHAPTER 2
**General Guidelines for Prescribing Therapeutic Plasma
    Exchange**   5
Kinetics of Immunoglobulin Removal   13

CHAPTER 3
Technique   18
Centrifugation   19
Filtration (Membrane Plasma Separation)   21
Therapeutic Plasma Exchange with Dialysis Equipment   23
    Operating Parameters   24
    Anticoagulation   25
    Vascular Access   25
Anticoagulation   26
Replacement Fluids   28
    Albumin   28
    Fresh Frozen Plasma   32
    Plasma Protein Fraction   34
    Starch Replacement for Therapeutic Plasma Exchange   35

Vascular Access 36
  Antecubital Veins 36
  Temporary Vascular Catheters 37
  Permanent Arteriovenous Access 41
Selective Plasmapheresis Techniques 42
  Cascade Filtration ("Double Filtration") 43
  Cryofiltration 45
  Immunoadsorbant Techniques 45
  Selective Lipid Removal 49
  Endotoxin Adsorption 52

CHAPTER 4
Complications and Management 53
Citrate-Induced Hypocalcemia 56
Coagulation Abnormalities 59
  "Depletion" Coagulopathy 59
  Thrombocytopenia 60
  Anemia 60
  Thrombosis 62
Infection 63
  Postpheresis Infection 64
  Risk of Viral Transmission 65
Reactions to Protein-Containing Replacement Fluids 69
Atypical Reactions Associated with Angiotensin-Converting
    Enzyme Inhibitors 71
Electrolyte Abnormalities 72
  Hypokalemia 72
  Alkalosis 72
  Aluminum 72
Vitamin Removal 73
Miscellaneous Complications 74
Hypotension 75
Deaths 76

CHAPTER 5
Drug Removal 78

PART II: Indications

CHAPTER 6
Introduction to Indications 85

CHAPTER 7
Neurologic Disorders   89
Guillain-Barré Syndrome   91
Myasthenia Gravis   94
Chronic Inflammatory Demyelinating Polyneuropathy   96
Paraprotein-Associated Polyneuropathy   98
Monoclonal Gammopathy of Undetermined Significance   98
Waldenström's Macroglobulinemia   98
Cryoglobulinemia   99
Multiple Sclerosis   100
Eaton-Lambert Syndrome   102
Stiff-Man Syndrome   103
Amyotrophic Lateral Sclerosis   104
Neuromyotonia (Isaacs' Syndrome)   105
Acute Disseminated Encephalomyelitis   105
Sensorineural Hearing Loss: Immune-Mediated Inner
     Ear Disease   106
Refsum's Disease   107

CHAPTER 8
Hematologic Disorders   110
Hyperviscosity Syndrome   110
Cryoglobulinemia   114
Thrombotic Thrombocytopenic Purpura   118
TTP in Pregnancy   122
HELLP Syndrome   123
HUS in Adults   125
HUS in Children   128
Idiopathic Thrombocytopenic Purpura   129
Post-Transfusion Purpura   133
Autoimmune Hemolytic Anemia   134
Cold Agglutinins   134
Warm Agglutinins   134
Maternal-Fetal Incompatibility: Rh Disease   136
Hemophilia: Removal of Factor VIII Inhibitors   137

CHAPTER 9
Metabolic Disorders   139
Hypercholesterolemia   139
Familial Hypercholesterolemia   140
Primary Biliary Cirrhosis   141
Hypertriglyceridemia   144

Pruritis Associated with Cholestasis   144
Hepatic Failure   145
Graves' Disease and Thyroid Storm   147
   Graves' Ophthalmopathy   148
Autoantibodies to the Insulin Receptor   149

CHAPTER 10
Dermatologic Disorders   151
Pemphigus Vulgaris   151
Bullous Pemphigoid   154
Toxic Epidermal Necrolysis (Lyell's Syndrome)   155
Porphyria Cutanea Tarda   156
Psoriasis   157

CHAPTER 11
Rheumatologic Disorders   159
Systemic Lupus Erythematosus   159
Lupus Anticoagulant, Anticardiolipin Antibodies, and the
   Antiphospholipid Antibody Syndrome   163
   Recurrent Fetal Loss   163
   Catastrophic Antiphospholipid Syndrome   164
   Renal Disease   164
Scleroderma   166
Rheumatoid Arthritis and Rheumatoid Vasculitis   169
   Rheumatoid Vasculitis   170
Vasculitis   172
Polymyositis and Dermatomyositis   175
Raynaud's Disease   176

CHAPTER 12
Renal Disease   178
Anti-GBM Antibody–Mediated Disease
   (Goodpasture's Syndrome)   180
Rapidly Progressive Glomerulonephritis   182
Renal Failure in Multiple Myeloma   186
IgA Nephropathy and Henoch–Schönlein Purpura   190
   Henoch-Schönlein Purpura   191
Focal Segmental Glomerulosclerosis: Recurrence
   Post-Transplant   192
Renal Allograft Rejection   193
The Transplant Candidate with Cytotoxic Antibodies   195

CHAPTER 13
**Indications for Therapeutic Plasma Exchange in the Intensive
    Care Unit** 197
Fulminant Systemic Meningococcemia 198
TPE for Septic Syndromes Other Than Meningococcemia 201
Burn Shock 205

CHAPTER 14
**Therapeutic Plasma Exchange in Patients with
    Human Immunodeficiency Virus** 206
General Comments 207
Risk of Accidental HIV Transmission to Patients and Staff 208
Immune Thrombocytopenic Purpura 209
Thrombotic Thrombocytopenic Purpura/Hemolytic Uremic
    Syndrome 209
Peripheral Neuropathy 210

CHAPTER 15
Intoxications 214
General Guidelines for the Use of TPE in the Treatment of
    Intoxications 215
Arsine 217
Carbamazepine 218
Cisplatin 218
Digitoxin Overdose 220
Digoxin-Specific Antibody Fragments 221
Diltiazem 221
Mushrooms: *Amanita phalloides* and *Amanita verna* 222
Mushrooms: Cortinarius 224
Mushrooms: *Paxillus involutus* 225
Paraquat Poisoning 225
Parathion Poisoning 226
Phenylbutazone 227
Phenytoin 227
Quinine 228
Sodium Chlorate Intoxication 229
Theophylline 229
Thyroxine 230
Tricyclic Antidepressants 230
Vincristine 232
Miscellaneous Intoxications 232

CHAPTER 16
Therapeutic Cytapheresis 234
Leukapheresis 234
  Leukapheresis for Hyperleukocytosis 235
  Lymphocytapheresis for Rheumatoid Arthritis 236
Thrombopheresis 237
Erythrocytapheresis 238
  Erythrocytapheresis for Sickle Cell Disease 238
  Erythrocytapheresis for Babesiosis 239
  Erythrocytapheresis for Falciparum Malaria 239

Index 241

List of Tables

TABLE 2-1
Estimated Plasma Volume by Weight and Hematocrit   6

TABLE 2-2
Distribution and Metabolism of Plasma Proteins   9

TABLE 3-1
Maximum Blood Flow Rates for Varying Ratios of Citrate Solution to Whole Blood   27

TABLE 3-2
ACD Anticoagulant Citrate Dextrose Solutions   28

TABLE 3-3
Protein A Immunoadsorption: Current and Potential Indications   46

TABLE 4-1
Complications of Plasmapheresis   54

TABLE 4-2
Calcium Kinetics with and without Supplemental Infusion   57

TABLE 4-3
Percent Decrease in Serum Levels of Coagulation Factors After a Single Plasma Exchange   59

TABLE 4-4
Risk of Transfusion-Transmitted Viral Infections per Unit Transfused in the Mid-1990s   66

TABLE 4-5
Potential Causes for Hypotension During TPE   76

TABLE 5-1
Drug Removal During Plasma Exchange   79

TABLE 5-2
Drugs with a High Percentage of Protein Binding and Modest
Volume of Distribution   80

TABLE 6-1
Indications for TPE   86

TABLE 7-1
Neurologic Indications for TPE   90

TABLE 7-2
The Guillain-Barré Syndrome Study Group: Controlled
Trial of TPE   92

TABLE 7-3
Observed and Predicted Decline in Anti-Acetylcholine Receptor
Antibody   95

TABLE 8-1
Hematologic Indications for TPE   111

TABLE 8-2
Controlled Trial of TPE vs. Plasma Infusion for TTP   119

TABLE 9-1
Metabolic Indications for TPE   140

TABLE 10-1
Dermatologic Indications for TPE   152

TABLE 11-1
Rheumatologic Indications for TPE   160

TABLE 11-2
Lymphopheresis and Plasmapheresis in Rheumatoid Arthritis   170

TABLE 12-1
Renal Indications for TPE   179

TABLE 12-2
Controlled Trials of TPE for Patients with Severe or
Dialysis-Dependent RPGN   184

TABLE 12-3
Controlled Study of TPE for the Treatment of "Cast
Nephropathy"   189

TABLE 13-1
Indications for TPE in the Intensive Care Unit   198

TABLE 13-2
TPE for Fulminant Meningococcemia   199

TABLE 13-3
Blood or Plasma Exchange for Patients with Sepsis/Septic Shock
(Excluding Meningococcemia)   202

TABLE 14-1
Indications for TPE in Patients with HIV   207

TABLE 15-1
TPE for Intoxications   215

TABLE 16-1
Therapeutic Cytapheresis   235

List of Figures

FIGURE 2-1
Percentage reduction in pretreatment serum concentrations versus the amount of volume exchanged   7

FIGURE 2-2
Immunoglobulin removal as a result of plasma exchange. Correlation between the predicted and actual percent decline in serum levels after a single TPE treatment   8

FIGURE 2-3
Progressive decline in pretreatment serum concentrations of IgG as a result of three consecutive plasma exchanges equaling one plasma volume each   10

FIGURE 2-4
Progressive decline in pretreatment serum concentrations of IgM as a result of three consecutive plasma exchanges equaling one plasma volume each   11

FIGURE 3-1
TPE with a continuous centrifugal system   20

FIGURE 3-2
Schematic section of a hollow fiber designed for TPE   21

FIGURE 3-3
Permeability of the Plasmaflo membrane   22

FIGURE 3-4
Circuitry for TPE with dialysis equipment   23

FIGURE 3-5
Plasma flow rate versus blood flow   24

FIGURE 4-1
Changes in PTT as a result of plasma exchange with
5% albumin   60

FIGURE 12-1
Light chains in serum and urine in a case of biopsy-proven "cast
nephropathy"   188

Preface

Once considered as little more than high-tech bloodletting, therapeutic plasma exchange (TPE) has been the subject of an increasing number of randomized, controlled studies that have better
defined its application for a wide variety of pathologic conditions.
Unfortunately, considering the relative rarity of the disease processes involved, the need for TPE treatment tends to be episodic
and it is difficult to remain familiar and current with the nuances
necessary to provide the most efficient and efficacious treatment
prescription. This book was created to provide a quick reference
guide to the practical application of TPE. Part I will cover the technical aspects of the treatment including a section describing the
kinetics of removing large-molecular-weight substances, a guide to
replacement fluids, and an exhaustive list of complications and their
management. Part II will deal with specific indications, where each
disease will be presented separately with an outline of treatment
rationale and a practical, reference-supported recommendation
regarding the amount and timing of the exchanges.

It is my hope that this volume will offer sufficient guidance
to aid any interested physician in providing a safe and efficacious
treatment for any disease process that may benefit from TPE.

A.A.K.

Operating Characteristics

Introduction and Rationale

1

Therapeutic plasma exchange (TPE) is an extracorporeal blood purification technique designed for the removal of large-molecular-weight substances. Examples of these substances include pathogenic autoantibodies, immune complexes, cryoglobulins, myeloma light chains, endotoxin, and cholesterol-containing lipoproteins. The basic premise of the treatment is that removal of these substances will reverse the pathologic processes related to their presence. Other potential benefits for TPE include an unloading of the reticuloendothelial system (1), stimulation of lymphocyte clones to enhance cytotoxic therapy (2), and the possibility of reinfusing large volumes of plasma without the risk of intravascular volume overload (3).

For TPE to be a rational choice as a blood purification technique, at least one of the following conditions should be met:

1. The substance to be removed is sufficiently large ($\geq$15,000 Da) so as to make other less-expensive purification techniques unacceptably inefficient (i.e., hemofiltration or high-flux dialysis).
2. The substance to be removed has a comparatively prolonged half-life, so that extracorporeal removal provides a therapeutically useful period of diminished serum concentration.
3. The substance to be removed is acutely toxic and resistant to conventional therapy, so that the rapidity of extracorporeal removal is clinically indicated.

The removal of pathogenic autoantibodies offers an example. If one considers that the natural half-life of IgG is approximately 21 days (4) and assuming that an immunosuppressive agent could immediately halt production (unlikely), the serum levels would

3

still be 50% of the initial values for at least 21 days after initiating therapy. Such a delay might be unacceptable in the presence of a very aggressive autoantibody such as that involved with Goodpasture's syndrome.

REFERENCES

1. Lockwood CM, Worlledge S, Nicholas A, Cotton C, Peters DK. Reversal of impaired splenic function in patients with nephritis or vasculitis (or both) by plasma exchange. N Engl J Med 1979; 300:524–530.
2. Schroeder JO, Euler HH, Loffler H. Synchronization of plasmapheresis and pulse cyclophosphamide in severe systemic lupus erythematosus. Ann Intern Med 1987;107:344–346.
3. Rock GA, Shumak KH, Buskard NA, Blanchette VS, Kelton JG, Nair RC, Spasoff RA. Comparison of plasma exchange with plasma infusion in the treatment of TTP. N Engl J Med 1991; 325:393–397.
4. Cohen S, Freeman T. Metabolic heterogeneity of human gamma globulin. Biochem J 1960;76:475–487.

General Guidelines for Prescribing Therapeutic Plasma Exchange

2

Kinetics of Immunoglobulin Removal   13

Specific prescription recommendations are given with each disease process (see specific chapters in Part II). This section offers guidelines on how to determine the amount of plasma to be exchanged during each treatment and how to space the treatments in a manner to provide the most efficient removal of a large-molecular-weight substance.

To prescribe therapeutic plasma exchange (TPE) in a rational manner, the amount of plasma to be exchanged must be determined in relation to the patient's estimated plasma volume (EPV). A simple means of estimating the EPV can be calculated from the patient's weight and hematocrit using the formula (1)

$$EPV = [0.065 \times wt(kg)] \times [1 - Hct] \tag{1}$$

where Hct equals hematocrit. This formula is one of many that have been proposed (2–5). It is offered in this volume because it directly relates the plasma volume estimate to the patient's hematocrit, it allows easy bedside calculation, and, in clinical use, it has provided a reliable prediction of overall treatment results (1,6). A rapid determination of the EPV for any given individual is provided in Table 2-1.

In general, large-molecular-weight substances (immunoglobulins, cholesterol-containing lipoproteins, cryoglobulins) are only slowly equilibrated between their extravascular and intravascular

**Table 2-1. Estimated Plasma Volume by Weight and Hematocrit:
EPV = [0.065 × wt (kg)] × [1 − Hct]**

		Hct%								
Wt (kg)	BV (L)	15	20	25	30	35	40	45	50	55
30	1.95	1.66	1.56	1.46	1.37	1.27	1.17	1.07	0.98	0.88
35	2.28	1.94	1.82	1.71	1.6	1.48	1.37	1.25	1.14	1.03
40	2.6	2.21	2.08	1.95	1.82	1.69	1.56	1.43	1.3	1.17
45	2.9	2.47	2.32	2.18	2.03	1.89	1.74	1.6	1.45	1.31
50	3.25	2.76	2.6	2.44	2.28	2.11	1.95	1.79	1.63	1.46
55	3.58	3.04	2.86	2.69	2.51	2.33	2.15	1.97	1.79	1.61
60	3.9	3.32	3.12	2.93	2.73	2.54	2.34	2.15	1.95	1.76
65	4.23	3.6	3.38	3.17	2.96	2.75	2.54	2.33	2.12	1.90
70	4.55	3.87	3.64	3.41	3.19	2.96	2.73	2.50	2.28	2.05
75	4.88	4.15	3.9	3.66	3.42	3.17	2.93	2.68	2.44	2.20
80	5.2	4.42	4.16	3.9	3.64	3.38	3.12	2.86	2.6	2.34
85	5.53	4.7	4.42	4.15	3.87	3.59	3.32	3.04	2.77	2.49
90	5.85	4.97	4.68	4.39	4.10	3.8	3.51	3.22	2.93	2.63
95	6.18	5.25	4.94	4.64	4.33	4.02	3.71	3.40	3.09	2.78
100	6.5	5.53	5.2	4.88	4.55	4.23	3.9	3.58	3.25	2.93
105	6.83	5.81	5.46	5.12	4.78	4.44	4.10	3.76	3.42	3.07
110	7.15	6.08	5.72	5.36	5.01	4.65	4.29	3.93	3.58	3.22
115	7.48	6.36	5.98	5.61	5.24	4.86	4.49	4.11	3.74	3.37
120	7.8	6.63	6.24	5.85	5.46	5.07	4.68	4.29	3.9	3.51
125	8.13	6.91	6.5	6.10	5.69	5.28	4.88	4.47	4.07	3.66
130	8.45	7.18	6.76	6.34	5.92	5.49	5.07	4.65	4.23	3.80
135	8.78	7.46	7.02	6.59	6.15	5.71	5.27	4.83	4.39	3.95
140	9.1	7.74	7.28	6.83	6.37	5.92	5.46	5.01	4.55	4.10

These values will not be valid for patients with severe hyperviscosity, such as in those with Waldenström's macroglobulinemia, in which plasma volumes will be greater than predicted (Bloch KJ, Maki DG. Hyperviscosity syndromes associated with immunoglobulin abnormalities. Semin Hematol 1973;20:113–124).

EPV values in liters. Wt, dry weight in kilograms; BV, blood volume in liters; Hct, hematocrit.

distribution. Thus, removal during a single treatment is essentially limited to that which is in the intravascular compartment and the amount of plasma to be exchanged to provide a given reduction in pretreatment levels can be determined by application of first-order kinetics using the formula

$$X_1 = X_0 e^{-V_e/\text{EPV}} \tag{2}$$

where X_1 equals the final plasma concentration, X_0 equals the initial concentration, V_e equals the volume exchanged, and EPV equals the patient's estimated plasma volume. The relation is plotted in

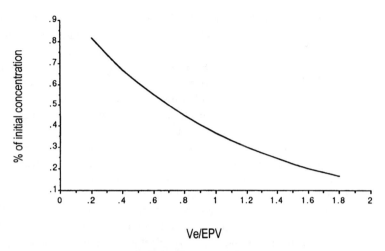

Figure 2-1. Percentage reduction in pretreatment serum concentrations versus the amount of volume exchanged. The volume exchanged (V_e) is plotted in relation to the patient's EPV. A single exchange equal to the patient's EPV (V_e/EPV = 1) will lower serum levels by approximately 63% and an exchange equal to 1.4 times the EPV (V_e/EPV = 1.4) will lower serum levels by 75%. Increasingly voluminous exchanges during a single treatment yield a progressively smaller reduction in pretreatment levels. (The percent reductions plotted on this graph are only valid for large-molecular-weight substances [immunoglobulins, lipoproteins, cryoglobulins, etc] that are slowly equilibrated between the extravascular and intravascular space. The plotted relation represents the formula $X_1 = X_0 e^{-V_e/EPV}$, where X_1 equals the final plasma concentration, X_0 equals the initial concentration, V_e equals the volume exchanged, and EPV equals the patient's estimated plasma volume; see text.)

Figure 2-1. For example, if the volume exchanged (V_e) is equal to the patient's EPV, pretreatment values will be lowered by 63%. If the plasma exchanged is equal to 1.4 times the EPV, the pretreatment levels will be lowered by 75%. As can be seen in Figure 2-1, increasingly voluminous exchanges during a single treatment yield a progressively smaller reduction in pretreatment levels. Given that overly voluminous exchanges will inefficiently increase the duration and costs of the treatment (i.e., replacement fluid and nursing time), for most indications, **each treatment should provide an exchange volume equaling 1 to 1.4 times the EPV.**

Clinical application and validation of the above calculations can be seen in Figure 2-2. The graphs demonstrate an excellent correlation between the predicted and actual percent decline in serum levels in each of the three immunoglobulin classes after a single TPE treatment. Of note is that the same type of correlation was found when these calculations were used to predict the decline in serum concentrations for cholesterol-containing lipoprotein and for the third component of complement (C3) (1).

It must be noted that the observed decline in serum concentrations of a given substance after a single TPE treatment bears little relation to the absolute decrease in total body load. Soon after the initial reduction in serum levels, there is a partial rebound. One component of this rebound represents a renewed synthesis of the substance, whereas another component is due to the extravascular to intravascular redistribution of the substance. Many large-molecular-weight substances, such as the immunoglobulins, have a substantial extravascular distribution Table 2-2 (7–19). After the rapid reduction in intravascular concentrations provided by the

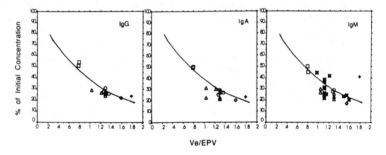

Ve/EPV

Figure 2-2. Immunoglobulin removal as a result of plasma exchange. Correlation between the predicted and actual percent decline in serum levels after a single TPE treatment. Predicted levels (solid line) were determined using first-order kinetics and assumed that the apparent volume of distribution was equal to the EPV. The abscissa represents the value V_e/EPV, where V_e equals the volume exchanged. The ordinate represents the final serum concentration as a percentage of the initial concentration. Correlation between the actual decline and predicated decline in serum values revealed an r value of 0.86 for IgG, 0.88 for IgA, and 0.57 for IgM. Several of the IgM levels were extremely low, at a point where measurements are less accurate. (Reproduced by permission from Kaplan AA, Halley SE. Plasma exchange with a rotating filter. Kidney Int 1990;38:160–166.)

TPE treatment, the extravascular distribution of the substance will re-equilibrate with the intravascular space. Considering that the extravascular distribution of a given substance cannot be removed until it has entered the intravascular space and considering that the extravascular to intravascular re-equilibration of a large–molecular-weight substance will be relatively slow (~1 to 3%/h), several consecutive treatments, separated by 24 to 48 hours each, will have to be performed to remove a substantial percentage of the total body burden. Examples of the progressive reduction in serum levels of

Table 2-2. Distribution and Metabolism of Plasma Proteins

Protein	Concentration (mg/mL)	M.W. × 10³ Da	Percent Intravascular	Fractional Turnover Rate (% day)	Half-life (days)
Normal physiology					
IgG (except IgG3 subclass)	12	150	45	7	22
IgG3	0.7	150	64	17	7
IgM[a]	0.9	950	78	19	5
IgA	2.5	160	42	25	6
IgD	0.02	175	75	37	2.8
IgE	0.0001	190	45	94	2.5
Albumin	45	66	44	11	17
C3	1.4	240	67	41	2
C4	0.5	200	66	43	2
Fibrinogen	3–4	340	81	24	4.2
Factor VIII	0.1	100–340	71	150	0.6
Antithrombin III	0.2	56–58	45	55	2.4
Lipoprotein cholesterol	1.5–2.0	1300	>90	—	3–5
Pathologic conditions					
Macroglobulinemia, IgM	50–130	950	89	25[a]	5.9
Bence Jones protein	4–10	10–25	<50	—[b]	—[b]
Endotoxin	$3–25 \times 10^{-7}$	100–2400[a]	>50	—[c]	—[c]
Immune complexes	—[a]	>300[a]	>50	—[c]	—[c]
TNF	$3–5 \times 10^{-7}$	50 (trimer)	<50		6–20 min

Values are averaged from those reported in the literature. Removal of a substance during a single TPE treatment is limited to that which is intravascular. Substances with substantial extravascular distribution require several consecutive TPE treatments to decrease total body burden. Those substances with short half-lives (high turnover rate) have a rapid return to pre-TPE levels unless production rates can be slowed by concomitant therapy.

[a] Highly variable or poorly defined.

[b] Highly dependent on degree of renal function, half-life greatly increased with renal failure.

[c] Half-life will be variable and dependent on the clearing capabilities of the reticuloendothelial system.

SOURCE: References 7–19.

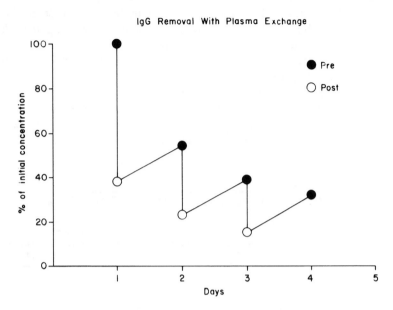

IgG Removal With Plasma Exchange

Figure 2-3. Progressive decline in pretreatment serum concentrations of IgG as a result of three consecutive plasma exchanges equaling one plasma volume each (V_e = EPV). Values plotted are the means of nine series of treatments in seven patients. The straight lines drawn between the post-treatment and pretreatment values are simplified representations of a complex curve that includes extravascular to intravascular redistribution and synthesis of a new antibody. The last value plotted was obtained 1 day after the third exchange, demonstrating a 70% decrease in pretreatment levels. (Reproduced by permission from Kaplan AA. Towards a rational prescription of plasma exchange: the kinetics of immunoglobulin removal. Semin Dial 1992;5:227–229.)

an immunoglobulin are given in Figures 2-3 and 2-4 (20). In general, if production rates (resynthesis) are modest (i.e., slowly forming antibody), at least **five separate treatments over a 7- to 10-day period will be required to remove 90% of the patient's initial total body burden** (20–24). If production rates are high (i.e., rapidly forming antibody, complement components), additional treatments may be required (25,26).

In conclusion, a rational approach to prescribing plasma exchange can be considered as follows: If the substance to be removed is measurable by reliable quantitative means, such as with a specific autoantibody, then the treatment schedule should be

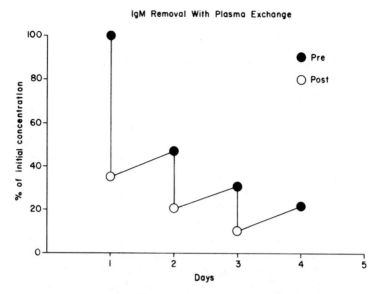

Figure 2-4.   Same as Figure 2-3, except for IgM. In contrast to the 70% decline plotted for IgG, the last value represents an approximate 80% reduction in total body burden, a reflection of the lesser extravascular distribution of the larger IgM molecule. (Reproduced by permission from Kaplan AA. Towards a rational prescription of plasma exchange: the kinetics of immunoglobulin removal. Semin Dial 1992;5:227–229.)

designed to achieve a substantial lowering of that substance using the kinetic considerations outlined above and taking into account the substance's rate of increase in the postpheresis period. If treatments are performed without identification of the offending agent, then the physician is dependent on empiric treatment schedules derived from the literature.

REFERENCES

1. Kaplan AA. A simple and accurate method for prescribing plasma exchange. Trans Am Soc Artif Intern Organs 1990;36: M597–M599.
2. Inkley SR, Brooks L, Krieger H. A study of methods for the prediction of plasma volume. J Lab Clin Med 1955;45: 841–850.

3. Retzlaff JA, Newlon Tauxe W, Kiely JM, Stroebel CF. Erythrocyte volume, plasma volume and lean body mass in adult men and women. Blood 1969;33:649–667.
4. Feldschuh J, Enson Y. Prediction of the normal blood volume: relation of blood volume to body habitus. Circulation 1977;56:605–612.
5. Sprenger KBG, Huber K, Kratz W, Henze E, Franz HE. Prediction of patient's plasma volume in plasma exchange therapy. In: Smeby LC, Jorstad S, Wideroe TE, eds. Immune and metabolic aspects of therapeutic blood purification systems. Basel: S. Karger, 1986:394–402.
6. Kaplan AA, Halley SE. Plasma exchange with a rotating filter. Kidney Int 1990;38:160–166.
7. Chopek M, McCullough J. Protein and biochemical changes during plasma exchange. In: Ulmas J, Berkman E, eds. Therapeutic hemapheresis: a technical workshop. Washington, DC: American Association of Blood Banks, 1980:13–52.
8. Morgenthaler JJ, Nydegger UE. Synthesis, distribution and catabolism of human plasma proteins in plasma exchange. Int J Artif Organs 1984;7:27–34.
9. Thornton CA, Griggs RC. Plasma exchange and intravenous immunoglobulin treatment of neuromuscular disease. Ann Neurol 1994;35:260–268.
10. Bowman BH. Hepatic plasma proteins: mechanisms of function and regulation. San Diego: Academic Press, Inc. Harcourt Brace Jovanovich, 1993.
11. Lockwood CM, Worlledge S, Nicholas A, Cotton C, Peters DK. Reversal of impaired splenic function in patients with nephritis or vasculitis (or both) by plasma exchange. N Engl J Med 1979;300:524–530.
12. Herbert LA. The clearance of immune complexes from the circulation of man and other primates. Am J Kidney Dis 1991;27:352–361.
13. Barth WF, Wochner D, Waldman TA, Fahey JL. Metabolism of human gamma macroglobulins. J Clin Invest 1964;43:1036–1048.
14. Russell JA, Fitzharris BM, Corringham R, Darcy DA, Powles RL. Plasma exchange v peritoneal dialysis for removing Bence Jones protein. Br Med J 1978;2:1397.
15. Fisher CJ Jr, Agosti JM, Opal SM, et al. Treatment of septic shock with the tumor necrosis factor receptor: Fc fusion protein. N Engl J Med 1996;334:1697–1702.

16. May ME, Mintz PD, Gray LS. Multicompartment analysis of the effects of plasmapheresis: application to lipid kinetics in humans. Am J Clin Pathol 1989;91:688–694.

17. Carter PW, Cohen HJ, Crawford J. Hyperviscosity syndrome in association with kappa light chain myeloma. Am J Med 1989;86:591–601.

18. Misiani R, Tiraboschi G, Mingardi G, Mecca G. Management of myeloma kidney: an anti-light chain approach. Am J Kidney Dis 1987;10:28–33.

19. Schetz M, Ferdinande P, Van den Berghe G, Verwaest C, Lauwers P. Removal of proinflammatory cytokines with renal replacement therapy: sense or non-sense? Intensive Care Med 1995;21:169–176.

20. Kaplan AA. Towards a rational prescription of plasma exchange: the kinetics of immunoglobulin removal. Semin Dial 1992; 5:227–229.

21. Roberts CG, Schindhelm K, Smeby LC, Farrell PC. Kinetic analysis of plasma separation: use of an animal model. In: Lysaght MJ, Gurland HJ, eds. Plasma separation and plasma fractionation. Basel: S. Karger, 1983:25–38.

22. Charlton B, Schindhelm K, Farrell PC. Effect of extracorporeal IgG removal on IgG kinetics. Trans Am Soc Artif Intern Organs 1983;29:724–729.

23. Kellogg RM, Hester JP. Kinetics modeling of plasma exchange: intra and post-plasma exchange. J Clin Apheresis 1988;4:183–187.

24. Keller AJ, Urbaniak SJ. Intensive plasma exchange on the cell separator: effects on serum immunoglobulins and complement components. Br J Haematol 1978;38:531–540.

25. Swainson P, Robson JS, Urbaniak SJ, Keller AJ, Kay AB. Treatment of Goodpasture's disease by plasma exchange and immunosuppression. Clin Exp Immunol 1978;32:233–242.

26. Jones JV, Robinson MF, Parciany RK, Layfer LF, McLeod B. Therapeutic plasmapheresis in systemic lupus erythematosus: effect on immune complexes and antibodies to DNA. Arthritis Rheum 1981;24:1113–1120.

KINETICS OF IMMUNOGLOBULIN REMOVAL

Specific recommendations for prescribing TPE for a particular indication are found in the appropriate chapter dealing with that disease (see Part II). This section provides the basis for an efficient prescription of TPE for the removal of immunoglobulins.

The basic tenets of immunoglobulin kinetics can be gleaned from the results of experiments in which isotopically labeled immunoglobulins have been infused into humans (1,2). These experiments have demonstrated that immunoglobulins have relatively long half-lives, approaching 21 days for IgG and 5 days for IgM; that immunoglobulins have a substantial extravascular distribution, approximately 60% for IgG and 20% for IgM; and that immunoglobulins exhibit an intravascular to extravascular equilibration that is relatively slow, approximating 1 to 3%/h (1–3).

Considering the relatively long half-lives of immunoglobulins, the use of immunosuppressive agents, which act only by depressing antibody synthesis, cannot be expected to substantially lower the levels of a pathogenic autoantibody for at least several weeks, even if production is completely blocked, hence the basic rationale for their removal by extracorporeal means. As detailed in the previous section, the relatively slow re-equilibration between the extravascular and intravascular compartment allows the use of first-order kinetics governing removal rates from a single compartment (i.e., the intravascular space). The calculations require that the volume exchanged (V_e) should be related to the volume of distribution of the substance from which it can be removed during the procedure, a volume that is limited to intravascular space and, for practical purposes, can be considered to be equal to the patient's EPV. An example of this exponential decline is given in the solid lines depicted in the three graphs of Figure 2-2. If the fraction V_e/EPV equals 0.7, the expected decrease will be 50%; if V_e equals EPV, the decrease should be 63%; and when V_e/EPV equals 1.4, the decrease should be 75%. Clinical validation of these predictions has been demonstrated for each major immunoglobulin class (see Figure 2-2) (4,5).

It must be noted that the observed decline in immunoglobulin levels after a single plasma exchange bears little relation to the absolute decrease in total body load. In effect, after a given TPE treatment, the extravascular distribution of an immunoglobulin will begin to enter the vascular space, yielding a posttreatment increase that will begin to level after 24 to 48 hours. After this re-equilibration, there will be a further opportunity for substantial removal of the immunoglobulin by a subsequent TPE treatment.

Using a mathematical model, Roberts et al (3) studied the kinetics of multiple plasma exchanges in rabbits. Their model predicts a 74% decline in total body load after three daily exchanges equaling one plasma volume each; the observed level was 69%. In close agreement with this animal data are our own observations obtained from nine series of treatments in seven patients. As seen in Figures 2-3 and 2-4, the expected re-equilibration after three daily exchanges yields an approximate 70% decline in total body load for IgG and an approximate 80% decline for IgM (6). Of note is that similar predictions can be made for other large-molecular-weight substances; however, extravascular to intravascular re-equilibration constants and overall serum half-lives should be known to perform the calculations (see Table 2-2) (7).

It should be kept in mind that the above-referenced calculations and the observed results describe a best-case scenario concerning immunoglobulin removal. In essence, these data are for an entire immunoglobulin class and not for any specific antibody. Although correlation between total IgG levels and pathogenic antibodies may be tightly correlated, such as with the relatively slowly produced antibody in myasthenia gravis (4) (see Table 7-3), in other autoimmune diseases, the rate of autoantibody production may greatly exceed that of the total immunoglobulin class. Such has been documented for certain cases of Goodpasture's syndrome where anti–glomerular basement membrane (GBM) anti-GBM activity is predictably lowered by a given plasma exchange treatment but for which the intertreatment increases in serum levels are too rapid to be compatible with a simple re-equilibration of extravascular stores (8). The same discordance has been documented in systemic lupus erythematosus, where, after extracorporeal removal by plasma exchange, anti-DNA binding activity may be produced at a far greater rate than that of the entire IgG class (9). Thus, a 70 to 80% absolute decrease in a pathogenic autoantibody requires at least three plasma exchange treatments and may require a far more intensive treatment schedule if production rates cannot be adequately controlled by the concomitant immunosuppressive medications.

Another potentially important factor that may necessitate a more extensive prescription of plasma exchange is the possibility of a post-treatment stimulation of pathogenic clones. Schroeder and Euler have reviewed the animal data and anecdotal human reports that suggested a stimulation of pathogenic antibody production after extracorporeal removal (10). These authors suggested that aggressive postpheresis immunosuppressive therapy may selectively target these activated pathogenic clones, thus producing a prolonged suppression of the autoantibody. Although the importance of this rebound phenomena has not been definitively demonstrated in humans, the available data are convincing enough to have stimulated an international study to determine the usefulness of postpheresis immunosuppression in cases of resistant lupus. Regardless of the results of this ambitious study, its design is of value because it underscores the importance of adding concomitant immunosuppressive therapy to any plasma exchange schedule designed to control an aggressive autoimmune disease.

REFERENCES

1. Cohen S, Freeman T. Metabolic heterogeneity of human gamma globulin. Biochem J 1960;76:475–487.
2. Barth WF, Wochner D, Waldmann TA, Fahey JL. Metabolism of human gamma macroglobulins. J Clin Invest 1964;43:1036–1048.
3. Roberts CG, Schindhelm K, Smeby LC, Farrell PC. Kinetic analysis of plasma separation: use of an animal model. In: Lysaght MJ, Gurland HJ, eds. Plasma separation and plasma fractionation. Basel: Karger, 1983:25–38.
4. Kaplan AA, Halley SE. Plasma exchange with a rotating filter. Kidney Int 1990;38:160–166.
5. Kaplan AA. A simple and accurate method for prescribing plasma exchange. Trans Am Soc Artif Intern Organs 1990;36:M597–M599.
6. Kaplan AA. Towards a rational prescription of plasma exchange: the kinetics of immunoglobulin removal. Semin Dial 1992;5:227–229.
7. Kellogg RM, Hester JP. Kinetics modeling of plasma exchange: intra and post-plasma exchange. J Clin Apheresis 1988;4:183–187.
8. Swainson P, Robson JS, Urbaniak SJ, Keller AJ, Kay AB. Treatment of Goodpasture's disease by plasma exchange and immunosuppression. Clin Exp Immunol 1978;32:233–242.
9. Jones JV, Robinson MF, Parciany RK, Layfer LF, McLeod B. Therapeutic plasmapheresis in systemic lupus erythematosus:

effect on immune complexes and antibodies to DNA. Arthritis Rheum 1981;24:1113–1120.

10. Schroeder JO, Euler HH, Loffler H. Synchronization of plasmaphereis and pulse cyclophosphamide in severe systemic lupus erythematosus. Ann Intern Med 1987;107:344–346.

Technique

3

Centrifugation   19
Filtration (Membrane Plasma Separation)   21
Therapeutic Plasma Exchange with Dialysis Equipment   23
   Operating Parameters   24
   Anticoagulation   25
   Vascular Access   25
Anticoagulation   26
Replacement Fluids   28
   Albumin   28
   Fresh Frozen Plasma   32
   Plasma Protein Fraction   34
   Starch Replacement for Therapeutic Plasma Exchange   35
Vascular Access   36
   Antecubital Veins   36
   Temporary Vascular Catheters   37
   Permanent Arteriovenous Access   41
Selective Plasmapheresis Techniques   42
   Cascade Filtration ("Double Filtration")   43
   Cryofiltration   45
   Immunoadsorbant Techniques   45
   Selective Lipid Removal   49
   Endotoxin Adsorption   52

Traditionally, plasma exchange was performed with centrifugation devices used in blood banking procedures. These devices offer the advantage of allowing for selective cell removal (cytapheresis) (1). Plasma exchange can also be performed with a highly permeable filter and standard dialysis equipment, a technique that is often referred to as membrane plasma separation (2). A detailed review of the available removal systems is provided by Sowada et al (3).

REFERENCES

1. Gurland HJ, Lysaght MH, Samtleben W, Schmidt B. A comparison of centrifugal and membrane based apheresis formats. Int J Artif Organs 1984;7:35–38.
2. Gurland HJ, Lysaght MJ, Samtleben W, Schmidt B. Comparative evaluation of filters used in membrane plasmapheresis. Nephron 1984;36:173–182.
3. Sowada K, Malchesky PS, Nose Y. Available removal systems: state of the art. In: Nydegger UE, ed. Therapeutic hemapheresis in the 1990s. Current Studies in Hematology and Blood Transfusion. Basel: Karger, 1990:51–113.

CENTRIFUGATION

Centrifugal systems for plasma exchange use G forces to separate the plasma into its different components (Fig 3-1). In increasing order of density (specific gravity, SG), whole blood constituents are layered into plasma (SG 1.025 to 1.029), platelets (1.040), lymph (1.070), granulocytes (1.087 to 1.092), and red cells (1.093 to 1.096). Separation of the plasma can be either intermittent or continuous. In the intermittent system, whole blood is collected into a receptacle (bowl) and centrifuged down to its plasma and cellular components. After separation, the cellular components are resuspended in an appropriate amount of replacement solution (i.e., albumin, fresh frozen plasma [FFP], etc.) and subsequently returned to the patient. The efficiency of this process is clearly limited by the amount of whole blood that can be safely removed from the patient, the extracorporeal volume (ECV). A device providing this type of intermittent separation is the Haemonetics V-50 (Haemonetics, Braintree, MA). Newer devices use a continuous flow system in which the whole blood is processed in an ongoing, online manner, allowing the ECV to be limited to that which is necessary for the blood tubing and the centrifugal receptacle. Most newer devices also offer several user-friendly modifications, including means for adjusting the amount of citrate anticoagulation (see Citrate-Induced Hypocalcemia, Chap. 4), automated control of blood flow and plasma separation, and volume regulation of the replacement fluid. In the United States and Canada, available continuous-flow devices include the Haemonetics MCS (Haemonetics, Braintree, MA), the Cobe Spectra (Cobe Laboratories, Lakewood, CO) and the Fresenius AS104 (Fresenius Medical

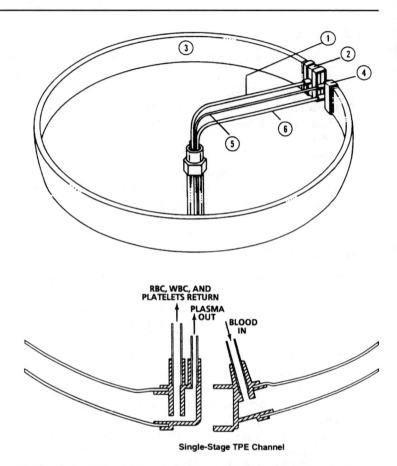

Single-Stage TPE Channel

Figure 3-1. TPE with a continuous centrifugal system. Anticoagulated blood enters the inlet chamber (2) through the inlet tube (1). As the channel (3) spins and the blood flows through the channel, the cellular components (platelets, WBCs, RBCs) settle toward the outside of the channel with the plasma on the inside. Most of the plasma is withdrawn through the "plasma out" tube, whereas all the cellular components exit through the "RBC return" tube. WBC, white blood cell; RBC, red blood cell. (Reproduced by permission from COBE SPECTRA Operator's Manual. Cobe BCT, Lakewood, CO.)

Care, Lexington, MA). A detailed review of the technical characteristics of these different machines has been published by Sawada et al (1). A basic video guide entitled Apheresis Instrumentation is available at modest cost from the **American Society for**

Apheresis (3900 East Timrod, Tuscon AZ 85711, telephone: 520-327-8584).

REFERENCE

1. Sowada K, Malchesky PS, Nose Y. Available removal systems: state of the art. In: Nydegger UE, ed. Therapeutic hemapheresis in the 1990s. Current Studies in Hematology and Blood Transfusion. Basel: Karger, 1990:51–113.

FILTRATION (MEMBRANE PLASMA SEPARATION)

Separation of plasma from the blood's cellular components can also be accomplished by filtration through a highly permeable membrane. This methodology separates the blood into its cellular and noncellular components by subjecting it to sieving through a membrane whose pores allow the plasma proteins to pass but that retain the larger cellular elements within the blood path (Figs 3-2 and 3-3). Pore sizes of these membranes are usually 0.6 µm or less, thus easily rejecting the smallest cellular component, the platelets (3 µm). Configuration of the semipermeable membrane can be in a layered flat plate design, such as is used in the Cobe Centry TPE (Cobe Laboratories, Lakewood, CO) (1); rolled in a tube, as used in the Fenwal Autopheresis C (Fenwal Laboratories, Deerfield, IL) (2,3);

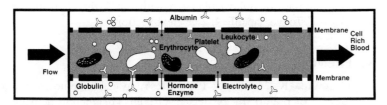

Figure 3-2. Schematic section of a hollow fiber designed for therapeutic plasma exchange. Whole blood flows lengthwise along the interior of the fiber, whereas its plasma components pass through the pores in the fiber wall and collect outside the fiber. The wall of the hollow fiber functions as the separating membrane with a pore size that allows penetration by plasma but not by the blood's cellular components (red and white blood cells, platelets). (Reproduced with permission from Apheresis Technologies, Palm Harbor, FL.)

21

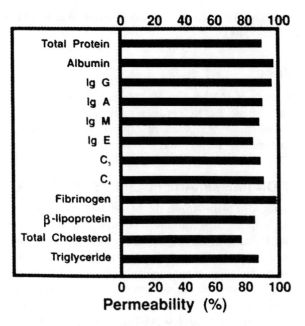

Figure 3-3. Permeability of the Plasmaflo membrane: Percentage sieving of large-molecular-weight proteins during TPE with the Plasmaflo membrane. Transmembrane pressure was maintained at 40 mm Hg and blood flow was at 100 mL/min. (Reproduced by permission from Apheresis Technologies, Palm Harbor, FL. Plasmaflo is a registered trademark of the Asahi Medical Co., LTD.)

or in bundles of hollow fibers, as with the Asahi Plasmaflo (Asahi Medical, Tokyo, Japan) (4) (see next section).

REFERENCES

1. Sowada K, Malchesky PS, Nose Y. Available removal systems: state of the art. In: Nydegger UE, ed. Therapeutic hemapheresis in the 1990s. Current Studies in Hematology and Blood Transfusion. Basel: Karger, 1990:51–113.
2. Kaplan AA, Halley SE, Reardon J, Sevigny J. One year's experience using a rotating filter for therapeutic plasma exchange. Trans Am Soc Artif Intern Organs 1989;35:262–264.
3. Kaplan AA. Two year clinical experience using a rotating filter for therapeutic plasma exchange. Proceedings of the World Apheresis Association, Amsterdam, 1990. In: Sibinga C, Kater L,

eds. Advances in haemapheresis. Dordrecht: Kluwer Academic Press, 1991:21–28.

4. Gurland HJ, Lysaght MJ, Samtleben W, Schmidt B. Comparative evaluation of filters used in membrane plasmapheresis. Nephron 1984;36:173–182.

THERAPEUTIC PLASMA EXCHANGE WITH DIALYSIS EQUIPMENT

When therapeutic plasma exchange (TPE) is performed with a highly permeable filter and standard dialysis equipment, it is often referred to as membrane plasma separation (MPS). Having undergone considerable investigation and use in both Europe and Japan (1,2), MPS has become increasingly popular in the United States. The highly permeable membrane, which is most often in a hollow fiber configuration, is connected to the blood pump and pressure monitoring system of the dialysis machine while the dialysis machine is used in its "isolated" ultrafiltration mode, which bypasses the dialysate proportioning system (Fig 3-4). Worldwide, there are

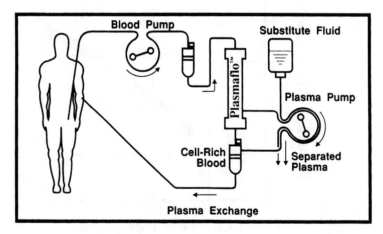

Figure 3-4. Circuitry for therapeutic plasma exchange with dialysis equipment. The plasma filter is placed in series in a manner to perform "isolated" ultrafiltration. The manufacturer of the Plasmaflo filter recommends that transmembrane pressure should be limited by the concomitant use of an additional roller pump to control the filtrate output rate. (Reproduced with permission from Apheresis Technologies, Palm Harbor, FL. Plasmaflo is a registered trademark of the Asahi Medical Co., LTD.)

a myriad of filters available for this purpose (2,3), but most are not available in the United States. The most commonly used membrane available in the United States is the cellulose diacetate Plasmaflo from Asahi Medical. In general, this filter can be used with any dialysis machine, but its blood tubing may be incompatible with the tubing path of some systems (i.e., the Cobe 3 and Hospal machines [Cobe Laboratories, Lakewood, CO]). Although thousands of these treatments are performed in the United States each year, the published American experience is very limited (4,5).

Operating Parameters

The Plasmaflo filter should be operated with a very modest transmembrane pressure (TMP) and blood flow (TMP <75 mm Hg, blood flows of 50 to 150 mL/min) to limit the tendency for hemolysis and filter clotting (Fig 3-5) (4,6). Limiting TMP can be most

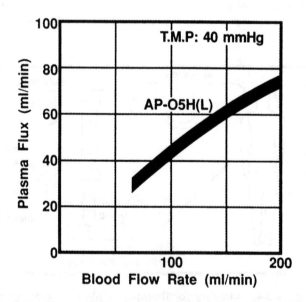

Figure 3-5.   Plasma flow rate versus blood flow. Plasma filtration rates of the Plasmaflo membrane at different blood flow rates. Transmembrane pressure was maintained at 40 mm Hg and blood flows varied from 40 to 200 mL/min. Hematocrit was between 30 and 40%. (Reproduced with permission from Apheresis Technologies, Palm Harbor, FL.)

easily achieved by limiting blood flows, but the filter's distributor recommends that treatments are performed with a double roller pump on the filtrate output of the filter (see Fig 3-4). This double pump is designed to appropriately limit the plasma flow rate and to regulate the infusion of replacement fluid (albumin, FFP, etc) by matching its rate of return to that of the plasma removed, thus eliminating the risk of hypotension or fluid overload. Of note is that protein permeable membranes such as the Plasmaflo are very susceptible to concentration polarization, a phenomenon whereby protein layering on the inner surface of the membrane rapidly limits the maximum achievable filtration rates (2). As a result, inappropriately high TMPs will not yield higher filtration rates but *will* increase the tendency for the filter to clog. There are several excellent reviews regarding the performance of MPS from a dialysis nursing perspective (6–8).

Anticoagulation

Most TPE treatments performed with centrifugal devices use citrate anticoagulation. Although this technique can be modified for use with an MPS system (9), most MPS treatments are performed with heparin. Initial recommendations are to start with a heparin dose of 5000 units (6) or 40–60 U/kg (4) and to follow with approximately 1000 U/h. Frasca et al (10) demonstrated that heparin doses should be increased with decreasing hematocrits and increasing plasma filtration rates, probably because of increasing volumes of distribution (with decreasing hematocrit) and increasing net removal (heparin was shown to have a sieving coefficient of 1 and therefore is removed more rapidly as filtration rates increase). It should be kept in mind that even when heparin is used for the system's anticoagulation, citrate toxicity is still possible if FFP is used as the replacement fluid, because FFP contains up to 14% citrate by volume (see Citrate-Induced Hypocalcemia, Chap. 4). This is most likely to occur when treating a patient with hepatic or renal failure (11). Ilamathi et al (9) reported the use of regional citrate anticoagulation for MPS using 22 mL/hr of citrate solution neutralized with 15 mL/hr of 10% calcium chloride solution.

Vascular Access

Because blood flow requirements are modest, TPE can be performed with any vascular access compatible with standard hemodialysis (see Vascular Access, below).

REFERENCES

1. Gurland HJ, Lysaght MH, Samtleben W, Schmidt B. A comparison of centrifugal and membrane based apheresis formats. Int J Artif Organs 1984;7:35–38.
2. Gurland HJ, Lysaght MJ, Samtleben W, Schmidt B. Comparative evaluation of filters used in membrane plasmapheresis. Nephron 1984;36:173–182.
3. Sowada K, Malchesky PS, Nose Y. Available removal systems: state of the art. In: Nydegger UE, ed. Therapeutic hemapheresis in the 1990s. Current Studies in Hematology and Blood Transfusion. Basel: Karger, 1990:51–113.
4. Gerhardt RE, Ntoso KA, Koethe JD, Lodge S, Wolf CJ. Acute plasma separation with hemodialysis equipment. J Am Soc Nephrol 1992;2:1455–1458.
5. Howard RL, Tatum K, Chan L, Shapiro JI. Performance of plasmapheresis by nephrologists: a survey. Dial Transpl 1990; 19:484.
6. Price CA. Therapeutic plasma exchange in a dialysis unit. ANNA J 1987;14:103–108.
7. Price CA, McCarley PB. Technical considerations of therapeutic plasma exchange as a nephrology nursing procedure. ANNA J 1993;20:41–46.
8. Price CA, McCarley PB. Physical assessment for patients receiving therapeutic plasma exchange. ANNA J 1994;21: 149–201.
9. Ilamathi E, Kirsch M, Moore B, Finger M. Citrate anticoagulation during plasmapheresis using standard hemodialysis equipment. Semin Dial 1993;6:268.
10. Frasca GM, Buscaroli A, Borgnino LC, Vangelista A. Optimization of heparin anticoagulation during membrane plasma separation. Int J Art Organs 1988;11:313–316.
11. Pearl RG, Rosenthal MH. Metabolic alkalosis due to plasmapheresis. Am J Med 1985;79:391–393.

ANTICOAGULATION

Regardless of the technique used, TPE normally requires some form of anticoagulation to avoid clotting within the extracorporeal circuit. For centrifugal techniques, this is often provided by citrate infusions that bind ionized calcium in the extracorporeal circuit such that the coagulation cascade is impeded. The ionized calcium level returns toward its original level as the blood is returned to the intravascular compartment where there are substantial stores of ionized calcium and where the citrate is metabolized. Nonetheless, signs of hypocalcemia ranging from circumoral paresthesias to QT prolongation of the electrocardiogram represent the most commonly reported secondary effects associated with TPE procedures (1,2). Thus, the goal of citrate anticoagulation is to provide enough to prevent clotting within the extracorporeal circuit while limiting the degree of systemic hypocalcemia resulting from the intravascular infusion of the citrate. In an indepth review of the subject, Hester et al (3) recommend that **citrate infusions should be limited to between 1.0 and 1.8 mg/kg/min**. Maintaining levels at, or below, 1.8 mg/kg/min can be roughly estimated by choosing a given ratio of citrate solution to whole blood and limiting the blood flows to a multiple of the patient's body weight. An example of this type of calculation is listed in Table 3-1. Clearly, however, these recommendations must be considered as general guidelines because of the extreme variability of a given patient to metabolize citrate, the possibility of pretreatment abnormalities in ionized calcium, and the variable content of citrate in the replacement solutions (FFP can contain up to 14% citrate by volume). If symptoms do occur, the same authors suggest calcium replacement with 10 mL of 10% calcium gluconate infused over 15 minutes approximately halfway through the procedure. Others believe that citrate toxicity can be reasonably well controlled with the oral administration of calcium tablets during the procedure, reserving intravenous calcium replacement only for those who develop symptoms. Solute content of representative citrate solutions is given in Table

Table 3-1. Maximum[a] Blood Flow Rates for Varying Ratios of Citrate Solution[b] to Whole Blood (WB)

ACD-A/WB	Maximum Flow Rate per kg Body Weight
1:10	$0.9 \times$ BW (kg)
1.15	$1.3 \times$ DW (kg)
1:20	$1.7 \times$ BW (kg)
1:25	$2.0 \times$ BW (kg)

[a] Assuming maximum citrate infusion of 1.8 mg/kg/min (see text).
[b] Formula ACD-A (Baxter, Deerfield, IL) (see Table 3-2).
BW, body weight.

Table 3-2. ACD Anticoagulant Citrate Dextrose Solutions*

	Concentrations
Formula A	
Dextrose	2.45 g/dL
Sodium citrate	2.2 g/dL
Citric acid	730 mg/dL
Total citrate	113 mmol/L
	21.3 mg/mL
Sodium concentration	252 mEq/L
Bicarbonate potential	336 mEq/L
Formula B	
Dextrose	1.47 g/dL
Sodium citrate	1.32 g/dL
Citric acid	440 mg/dL
Total citrate	73 mmol/L
	14 mg/mL
Sodium concentration	150 mEq/L
Bicarbonate potential	219 mEq/L

*Baxter, Deerfield, IL.

3-2. (For a more detailed discussion regarding citrate toxicity, see Chap. 4.)

REFERENCES

1. Mokrzycki MH, Kaplan AA. Therapeutic plasma exchange: complications and management. Am J Kidney Dis 1994;23: 817–827.
2. Olson PR, Cox C, McCullough J. Laboratory and clinical effects of the infusion of ACD solution during platelet-pheresis. Vox Sang 1977;33:79–87.
3. Hester JP, McCullough J, Mishler JM, Szymanski IO. Dosage regimens for citrate anticoagulants. J Clin Apheresis 1983; 1:149–157.

REPLACEMENT FLUIDS
Albumin

General comments: Albumin is the most commonly used replacement fluid in the United States and, when compared with FFP, has the advantage of lacking viral transmission and possessing a decreased risk of anaphylactoid reactions. Disadvantages include a post-treatment coagulopathy related to the removal of clotting factors and a net loss of immunoglobulins. A 5% concentration of albumin provides a reasonable replacement of the oncotic pressure removed with the patient's plasma (see below). Some centers prefer to dilute the albumin to approximately 3.5%, a solution that is hypo-oncotic to the plasma that is being removed and may render the patient more prone to hypotension.

Colloid oncotic pressure: In a study that measured colloid oncotic pressure, 5% albumin was found to be slightly hypo-oncotic to the patients' plasma (18 versus 22 torr), but at least one of the patients studied had a condition in which oncotic pressure would be abnormally high (Waldenström's macroglobulinemia) (1). In contrast, Chopek and McCullough (2) demonstrated a slight hemodilution effect occurring after replacement with 5% albumin, suggesting that, in clinical use, this solution is slightly hyperoncotic and may result in mild intravascular expansion. McLeod et al (3) studied the use of partial albumin replacement using a replacement schedule involving 750 mL of saline followed by 1250 mL of 5% albumin. They found this combination to be well tolerated and no patient developed hypotension or peripheral edema, but the exchanges were limited to 2 liters, a rather modest volume for most TPE prescriptions.

Electrolyte composition: Five percent human serum albumin is isosmotic to plasma, contains no preservatives, and is characterized by a sodium level of approximately 145 ± 15 mmol/L and a potassium level lower than 2 mmol/L (4). The relative lack of potassium can result in a 25% reduction of serum potassium levels in the immediate postpheresis period, leading to a risk of hypokalemic arrhythmia (a situation most likely to occur in patients taking digitalis preparations). This type of postpheresis hypokalemia can be avoided by adding 4 mmol of potassium to each liter of 5% albumin.

Albumin solutions are contaminated with between 4 and 24 mmol/L of aluminum (5,6), and massive replacement with albumin may result in aluminum accumulation (see Electrolyte Abnormalities, Chap. 4).

Anaphylactic reactions: Human serum albumin consists of 96% albumin and trace amounts of alpha and beta globulins and, as opposed to FFP, anaphylactoid reactions are rare and may be associated with the formation of antibodies to polymerized albumin created by heat treatment or stabilization with sodium caprylate (4,7,8). Recent reports suggested that patients taking angiotensin-converting enzyme (ACE) inhibitors may also be prone to increased risk of "atypical" or hypotensive reactions to albumin (9,10) (see Reactions to Protein-Containing Replacement Fluids and Atypical Reactions Associated with ACE Inhibitors, Chap. 4).

Depletion coagulopathy: When albumin is used as the sole replacement fluid, there is a depletion of all coagulation factors. After a single plasma exchange, prothrombin time increases approximately 30% and partial thromboplastin time doubles (11). Although there is variability among patients, especially when clotting factor production may be compromised (liver failure), partial thromboplastin time and thrombin time return toward the normal range in approximately 4 hours, whereas prothrombin time normalizes in 24 hours (12). When multiple treatments are performed over a short period (i.e., three or more treatments per week), the depletion in clotting factors is more pronounced and may require several days for spontaneous recovery (12,13). Under these conditions, the risks of hemorrhage can be minimized with a partial replacement of FFP given toward the end of the procedure (see Coagulation Abnormalities, Chap. 4).

Immunoglobulin depletion: When albumin is used as the replacement fluid, removal of immunoglobulins and complement may predispose patients to high rates of infection. One plasma volume exchange results in a 60% reduction in serum immunoglobulin levels and a net 20% reduction in total body immunoglobulin stores (9) (see Kinetics of Immunoglobulin Removal, Chap. 2). Multiple treatments over short periods, especially when associated with immunosuppressive agents, yield a substantial decrease in immunoglobulin levels that may persist for several weeks (14–16). If serious infection occurs soon after a series of TPE treatments, a one time infusion of intravenous immunoglobulin (IVIG) at 100 to 400 mg/kg will reconstitute normal immunoglobulin levels (see Infection, Chap. 4).

Risk of viral transmission: Albumin preparations are treated with heat and are considered to be devoid of transmissible virus (4). The same claims were made for IVIG (17), but an outbreak of hepatitis C from contaminated IVIG has been documented (18) and new methodologies for avoiding viral transmission from IVIG preparations have been initiated (19).

REFERENCES

1. Lasky LC, Finnerty EP, Genis L, Polesky HF. Protein and colloid osmotic pressure changes with albumin and/or saline replacement during plasma exchange. Transfusion 1984;24: 256–259.
2. Chopek M, McCullough J. Protein and biochemical changes during plasma exchange. In: Ulmas J, Berkman E, eds. Therapeutic hemapheresis: a technical workshop. Washington, DC: American Association of Blood Banks, 1980:13–52.
3. McLeod BC, Sassetti RJ, Stefoski D, Davis FA. Partial plasma protein replacement in therapeutic plasma exchange. J Clin Apheresis 1983;1:115–118.
4. Finlayson JS. Albumin products. Semin Thromb Hemost 1980; 6:85–120.
5. Mousson C, Charhon SA, Ammar M, Accominotti M, Rifle G. Aluminum bone deposits in normal renal function patients after long-term treatment by plasma exchange. Int J Artif Organs 1989;23:664–667.
6. Milliner DS, Shinaberger JH, Shurman P, Coburn JW. Inadvertent aluminum administration during plasma exchange due to aluminum contamination of albumin replacement solutions. N Engl J Med 1985;312:165–167.
7. Apter AJ, Kaplan AA. An approach to immunologic reactions with plasma exchange. J Allergy Clin Immunol 1992;90: 119–124.
8. Stafford CT, Lobel SA, Fruge BC, Moffitt JE, Hoff RG, Fadel HE. Anaphylaxis to human serum albumin. Ann Allergy 1988; 61:85–88.
9. Brecher ME, Owen HG, Collins ML. Apheresis and ACE inhibitors. Transfusion 1993;33:963–964. Letter.
10. Owen HG, Brecher ME. Atypical reactions associated with use of angiotensin-converting enzyme inhibitors and apheresis. Transfusion 1994;34:891–894.

11. Kaplan AA, Halley SE. Plasma exchange with a rotating filter. Kidney Int 1990;38:160–166.
12. Chrinside A, Urbaniak SJ, Prowse CV, Keller AJ. Coagulation abnormalities following intensive plasma exchange on the cell separator. Br J Haematol 1981;48:627–634.
13. Mokrzycki MH, Kaplan AA. Therapeutic plasma exchange: complications and management. Am J Kidney Dis 1994;23: 817–827.
14. Kaplan AA. Towards a rational prescription of plasma exchange: the kinetics of immunoglobulin removal. Semin Dial 1992;5: 227–229. Editorial.
15. Sultan Y, Bussel A, Maisonneuve P, Sitty X, Gajdos P. Potential danger of thrombosis after plasma exchange in the treatment of patients with immune disease. Transfusion 1979;19: 588–593.
16. Keller AJ, Urbaniak SJ. Intensive plasma exchange on the cell separator. Effects on serum immunoglobulins and complement components. Br J Haematol 1978;38:531–540.
17. Haas A. Use of intravenous immunoglobulin in immunoregulatory disorders. In: Stiehm ER, moderator. Intravenous immunoglobulins as therapeutic agents. Ann Intern Med 1987; 107:367–382.
18. Bjoro K, Froland SS, Yun Z, Samdal HH, Haaland T. Hepatitis C infection in patients with primary hypogammaglobulinemia after treatment with contaminated immune globulin. N Engl J Med 1994;331:1607–1611.
19. Schiff RI. Transmission of viral infections through intravenous immune globulin. N Eng J Med 1994;331:1649–1650. Editorial.

Fresh Frozen Plasma

General comments: FFP contains all the noncellular components of normal blood and does not lead to postpheresis coagulopathy nor immunoglobulin depletion. FFP is also considered essential for the treatment of thrombotic thrombocytopenic purpura (TTP) because TPE for this indication may be most useful as a means of providing a missing serum factor (1) (see section on TTP/HUS in Chap. 8). Disadvantages include anaphylactoid reactions (most often mild but can be life threatening), citrate toxicity, and a small but persistent risk of viral transmission. Because of these potential problems, FFP should be avoided except for the treatment of TTP hemolytic uremia syndrome (HUS) or when hemorrhagic risks are great.

Anaphylactoid reactions: Anaphylactoid reactions to FFP are common and have been reported to occur with an incidence of up to 21% (2) (see Table 4-1). Symptomatology may vary and includes fever, rigors, urticaria, wheezing, and hypotension (3,4). These reactions are among the most serious encountered during TPE procedures, and the uncommon reports of TPE-related deaths are most often associated with FFP replacement (5–8). Because these reactions may involve the formation of kinins, the use of ACE inhibitors should be avoided in patients undergoing TPE (see more detailed discussion in Reactions to Protein-Containing Replacement Fluids and Atypical Reactions Associated with ACE Inhibitors, Chap. 4).

Because of the relative high incidence of these reactions, patients undergoing massive replacement with FFP (for TTP or HUS) are commonly pretreated with 50 mg of diphenhydramine. In those patients who have already demonstrated a sensitivity to FFP, we recommend oral dosing of 50 mg of prednisone given 13, 7, and 1 hour before the treatment, combined with 50 mg of diphenhydramine and 25 mg of ephedrine given 1 hour before the treatment (9). **In the event of a severe life-threatening reaction (laryngeal edema, etc), 0.3–0.5 mL of epinephrine (1:1000 solution) should be available for subcutaneous administration.**

Citrate toxicity: FFP contains approximately 14% citrate by volume, and large infusions of FFP may lead to symptoms of hypocalcemia and metabolic alkalosis. Symptoms of hypocalcemia can be avoided with the prophylactic replacement of calcium. Metabolic alkalosis, most common in patients with severe renal failure, may require concomitant hemodialysis (2,10). In this regard, those patients requiring TPE with FFP replacement who are also undergoing hemodialysis (TTP/HUS, Goodpasture's syndrome postbiopsy, etc) should be hemodialysed *after* the TPE treatment to facilitate correction of the citrate-induced alkalemia (see Citrate-Induced Hypocalcemia, Chap. 4).

Risk of viral transmission: Risk of viral transmission during plasma exchange is directly related to replacement with FFP. The current incidence of transfusion-acquired viral infections has declined substantially from the early 1980s and is currently estimated as 1 in 63,000 units for hepatitis B, 1 in 100,000 units for hepatitis C, 1 in 680,000 units for human immunodeficiency virus, and 1 in 641,000 units for human T-cell lymphotropic virus (11–13). It should be noted that during a single plasma volume exchange with FFP (~3 liters), 10–15 units, obtained from an equal number of donors, are used (see Infection, Chap. 4).

Plasma Protein Fraction

Plasma protein fraction (PPF) contains approximately 87% albumin and 13% alpha and beta globulins and is easier and less costly to prepare than albumin. Although difficult to prove, the risk of anaphylactoid reaction is probably less than for that of FFP (see above). Nonetheless, PPF has been associated with hypotensive episodes and circulatory collapse, possibly due to the presence of prekallikrein activator and bradykinin (14). As with the use of FFP, concomitant treatment with ACE inhibitors should be avoided.

REFERENCES

1. Rock GA, Shumak KH, Buskard NA, Blanchette VS, Kelton JG, Nair RC, Spasoff RA, and the Canadian Apheresis Study Group. Comparison of plasma exchange with plasma infusion in the treatment of TTP. N Engl J Med 1991;325: 393–397.
2. Mokrzycki MH, Kaplan AA. Therapeutic plasma exchange: complications and management. Am J Kidney Dis 1994;23: 817–827.
3. Ring J, Messmer K. Incidence and severity of anaphylactoid reactions to colloid volume substitutes. Lancet 1977;1: 466–469.
4. Bambauer R, Jutzler GA, Albrecht D, Keller HE, Kohler M. Indications of plasmapheresis and selection of different substitution solutions. Biomater Artif Cells Artif Organs 1989;17: 9–27.
5. Huestis DW. Mortality in therapeutic haemapheresis. Lancet 1983;1:1043. Letter.
6. Aufeuvre JP, Morin-Hertel F, Cohen-Solar M, Lefloch A, Baudelot J. Hazards of plasma exchange. In: Sieberth HG, ed. Plasma exchange. Stuttgart, Germany: FK Schattauer Verlag, 1980:149–157.

7. Aufeuvre JP, Mortin-Hertel F, Cohen-Solal M, Lefloch A, Baudelot J. Clinical tolerance and hazards of plasma exchanges: a study of 6200 plasma exchanges in 1033 patients. In: Beyer JH, Burgerg H, Fuchs C, Nagel GA, eds. Plasmapheresis in immunology and oncology. Basel, Switzerland: Karger, 1982: 65–77.

8. Sutton DMC, Nair R, Rock G, and the Canadian Apheresis Study Group. Complications of plasma exchange. Transfusion 1989;29:124–127.

9. Apter AJ, Kaplan AA. An approach to immunologic reactions with plasma exchange. J Allergy Clin Immunol 1992;90: 119–124.

10. Pearl RG, Rosenthal MH. Metabolic alkalosis due to plasmapheresis. Am J Med 1985;79:391–393.

11. Lackritz EM, Satten GA, Aberle-Grasse J, Dodd RY, Raimondi VP, Janssen RS, et al. Estimated risk of transmission of the human immunodeficiency virus by screened blood in the United States. N Engl J Med 1995;333:1721–1725.

12. Schreiber GB, Busch MP, Kleinman SH, Korelitz JJ. The risk of transfusion-transmitted virus infections. The Retrovirus Epidemiology Donor Study. N Engl J Med 1996;334: 1685–1690.

13. AuBuchon JP, Birkmeyer JD, Busch MP. Safety of the blood supply in the United States: opportunities and controversies. Ann Intern Med 1997;127:904–909.

14. Finlayson JS. Albumin products. Semin Thromb Hemost 1980; 6:85–120.

Starch Replacement for Therapeutic Plasma Exchange

Product shortages and rising costs may necessitate the use of non-protein-containing solutions as replacement fluids for TPE. Recently, Owen and Brecher have investigated the use of hydroxyethyl starch (Hespan; DuPont, Wilmington, DE) as a partial or full replacement for albumin (1–3). This starch-based colloid solution is biochemically similar to glycogen, rendering it unlikely to engender immune reactions. In one study, 7 patients received 1000 mL of 6% hetastarch as part of their replacement fluid during 33 procedures, whereas a further 42 patients received 1000 mL of 3% hetastarch during 289 procedures (2). In those receiving 3% hetastarch, the blood pressure and pulse remained stable for 97.3% of the procedures (280 treatments). Two patients receiving the 6% solution and one in the 3% group complained of severe transient back and head pain during hetastarch infusion. Total protein decreased in both groups, but only one patient reported slight peripheral edema after two procedures, suggesting a modest decline in serum oncotic pressure. The authors concluded that 3% hetastarch was a safe and cost-effective partial replacement for albumin during TPE. Kinetic modeling of the washout of starch used as a replacement fluid demonstrated that relatively little residual starch remains compared with the total amount infused (3). As an example, if six successive 4-liter exchanges were performed using only starch as the replacement solution, only 4.1 liters of starch (4 liters × six exchanges × 17% = 4.1 liters) would be expected to remain in the circulation despite a total infusion of 24 liters (4 liters × six exchanges = 24 liters) of starch.

REFERENCES

1. Brecher ME, Owen HG, Bandarenko N. Alternatives to albumin: starch replacement for plasma exchange. J Clin Apheresis 1997;12:146–153.
2. Owen HG, Brecher ME. Partial colloid starch replacement for therapeutic plasma exchange. J Clin Apheresis 1997;12:87–92.
3. Brecher ME, Owen HG. Washout kinetics of colloid starch as a partial or full replacement for plasma exchange. J Clin Apheresis 1996;11:123–126.

VASCULAR ACCESS
Antecubital Veins

Under ideal circumstances, vascular access can be provided by bilateral cannulation of the antecubital veins. When possible, this approach is clearly the safest and most desirable. On the negative side, the treatments may be unnecessarily prolonged because blood flows may be limited; the patient is incapacitated throughout the entire treatment, with no use of either arm; and the patient will commonly have to perform repeated exercise of the hands to stimulate flow, thus necessitating continued vigilance and cooperation. If the treatments are scheduled in advance or are being performed on a regular interval, the patient should be instructed to perform hand exercises to stimulate blood flow and promote venous dilatation. Repetitive squeezing of a tennis ball is often useful.

When the antecubital venous approach is not possible or practical, there are two types of alternatives: the use of a **percutaneous or implanted catheter** or the surgical placement of a permanent **arteriovenous fistula or graft**. Both entail their own risks and benefits and are discussed separately. In general, they both have the advantage of allowing the most efficient treatments by providing high blood flows and requiring minimal cooperation from the patient during the procedure. The percutaneous catheters are best used when there is the expectation for a limited number of treatments to be performed, such as might be used for the management of Guillain-Barré syndrome. Another common scenario would be to use this access in a critically ill patient when TPE is being performed concurrently with hemodialysis, such as might occur with autoimmune glomerulonephritis or the hemolytic uremic syndrome. The permanent arteriovenous accesses, commonly used for maintenance hemodialysis, are best reserved for those patients in whom repeated treatments are expected over a prolonged period, such as might be used for the management of familial hypercholesterolemia or chronic demyelinating polyneuropathies. The implanted catheters provide a compromise between these two extremes, allowing a more prolonged access (weeks or months) than the percutaneous catheters without the need for the permanent vascular surgery required for an arteriovenous fistula or graft.

Temporary Vascular Catheters

Infection control: Ideally, these catheters should not be used for any other purpose other than the TPE treatment itself. Exit sites should be maintained with meticulous care. Many centers have well-defined protocols that involve the use of povidone-iodine ointment and a sterile occlusive dressing (1). The dressing should be changed after each use and the exit site inspected for erythema or purulence. Unexplained fever (>38°C) should alert the physician to the possibility of catheter infection, even if the exit site appears unaffected. If no other source of infection can be identified (history, physical, chest x-ray, urinalysis), up to 50% may have catheter colonization, 35% will have catheter sepsis, and 20% will have sepsis from another source (1), results that argue strongly for catheter removal. Positive blood cultures taken through the access ports may help to document the catheter as the site of infection (see below). If an alternative site of infection is identified and there is no obvious sign of infection at the catheter exit site, the distal site can be treated while awaiting the results of blood cultures drawn through the catheter. Catheters removed for suspected infection should be cultured by cutting the distal 5 cm (intravenous portion) of the catheter with sterile scissors. The resulting catheter tip should be sent to the bacteriology laboratory in a sterile container. Catheter sepsis is defined when both the catheter tip and the blood cultures drawn through the catheter grow the same organism. Alternatively, if the blood cultures grow an organism not found on culture of the catheter tip, a noncatheter origin of the infection should be suspected. Using the technique of Maki et al (2) (using agar plates rather than broth), subclinical catheter infection or colonization in the afebrile patient can be defined when the catheter tip grows greater than 15 colonies of bacteria, whereas those tips yielding growth of less than 15 colonies may be considered to have been contaminated during removal. Most catheter-related infections are with *Staphylococcus aureus* or *S. epidermidis*. *Candida* species, *Streptococcus* species, and gram-negative organisms have also been implicated. Of note are the results of two recent studies suggesting that catheters impregnated with either a combination of rifampin and minocycline (3) or chlorhexidine and silver sulfadiazine (4) were less likely to become infected.

Maintaining patency: If the catheter is to be used for a subsequent treatment, the likelihood of intertreatment catheter clotting can be minimized by the instillation of 1 mL of 10,000 U/mL heparin solution into each catheter port (5). Catheter clotting is not infrequent and may respond to a heparin or saline flush. If there is no evidence for infection, a malfunctioning or clotted percutaneous catheter may be replaced over a guidewire, a procedure that has not been associated with a higher infection rate (1). Catheter clotting may also respond to instillation of urokinase. A solution of urokinase (5000 IU/mL) is gently injected into the catheter in a volume to approximate the internal volume of the catheter (often 1 to 1.5 mL) so that it can reach the catheter's tip without entering the systemic circulation. Aspiration can be attempted after 5 to 20 minutes. If repeated attempts are unsuccessful, a second injection of urokinase can be attempted (5). Alternatively, recombinant tissue-type plasminogen activator (rt-PA) can be used. In one successful application, a solution of 50 mg of rt-PA (29,000 IU) was mixed with 50 mL of 0.9% saline and infused into one lumen of the catheter over 4 hours (6). rt-PA has the advantage of being nonantigenic and is only activated in the presence of fibrin, thus being less likely to cause systemic hemorrhage.

Of note is that removal of a large-bore double-lumen catheter may be particularly hazardous after an intensive run of TPE treatments using albumin replacement, a situation that will result in a substantial "depletion" coagulopathy (7). Under these conditions, it may be useful to allow the catheter to remain in situ until there is a natural return of normal clotting parameters (prothrombin time, partial thromboplastin time). If the catheter must be removed immediately after a TPE treatment, 500 mL to 1 liter of FFP should be substituted as the replacement solution toward the end of the treatment to minimize the hemorrhagic risk (see Coagulation Abnormalities, Chap. 4).

In general, catheters intended for the infusion of chemotherapy (i.e., small-bore Hickman catheters) are not suited for providing the necessary blood flow for an efficient TPE treatment.

Femoral vein cannulation: The percutaneous placement of a double-lumen catheter in the femoral vein is the most widely used method for obtaining access to the central venous circulation. Extensive experience in its use for acute hemodialysis has found this method to be safe and well tolerated, despite repeated punctures. A disadvantage is that the catheter strongly limits the patient's mobility and is best suited for the bedridden. For TPE, this method is most useful for a relatively short and defined treatment schedule, such as might be used for the treatment of acute exacerbations of myasthenia gravis or the removal of light chains in multiple myeloma. An unresolved issue is the length of time that a single catheter can be safely left in place. Ideally, the catheter should be removed after every procedure; however, this is often impractical or impossible. In any event, catheters should never be left in situ for more than several days, and removed catheter tips should be sent for culture (see above). Careful attention to sterility during placement and meticulous access site care are essential. The most serious complications include retroperitoneal hemorrhage and pulmonary embolus. Retroperitoneal hemorrhage may result from iliac vein rupture and has been associated with difficult guidewire placement. Pulmonary emboli are the result of catheter-related thrombi and are most likely to occur with catheters left in situ for prolonged periods. Other complications include hematomas, thrombophlebitis, arteriovenous fistulae, sepsis, and access site infection (8).

Subclavian catheters: This access allows unhindered patient mobility and has been safely left in place for several weeks. Its major disadvantage is that it is associated with an increased risk of life-threatening complications. **Radiologic evaluation for catheter placement is required before the first treatment.** Sharp angulations of the distal catheter tip necessitate catheter repositioning to avoid vessel rupture. Massive hemothorax and pericardial tamponade are among the most serious complications. Particularly troublesome is that these complications can occur even after previously successful treatments. Arrhythmias, thrombophlebitis, sepsis, air embolism, pneumothorax, and access site infection are other complications (9,10). It is also well established that prolonged cannulation can lead to significant subclavian venous stenosis, thus rendering the ipsilateral arm incapable of supporting permanent angioaccess (11). Because of this risk of stenosis, this access should be avoided in any patient in whom there is an anticipated possibility for the need of permanent subcutaneous access, such as with a patient with renal failure or with familial hypercholesterolemia.

Internal jugular catheters: The internal jugular approach offers an alternative to subclavian cannulation. A potential advantage to this method is that the catheter's position is relatively straight, thus avoiding the sharp angulations associated with the subclavian route (12). Nonetheless, retrograde cannulation of the subclavian vein is possible, and **radiologic evaluation of placement is required**. A drawback to this technique is the relatively awkward placement and the difficulty of access site care. Subcutaneous tunneling of the catheter exit site may lower the incidence of infection (13).

Tunneled jugular venous catheters (PermCath): The PermCath (Quinton Instruments Company, Seattle, WA) is a highly pliable Dacron catheter that requires surgical placement but combines the safety of the jugular venous route (little risk of intravascular or intracardiac puncture) and the convenience of the subclavian percutaneous exit site. This catheter offers a more prolonged "temporary" access site that can be used for weeks or months (5). Choice of this type of access is best suited for an intermediate duration of treatment. In one case, we used this access in a pregnant patient requiring several months of TPE treatments for TTP.

Permanent Arteriovenous Access

These surgically created vascular fistulas are those most commonly used to provide hemoaccess for chronic maintenance hemodialysis (14). In general, this type of permanent vascular access is not commonly warranted in the patient requiring TPE. Exceptions are in patients whose treatments may be repeated on a prolonged or semipermanent basis, such as those being treated for familial hypercholesterolemias or those with chronic demyelinating inflammatory polyneuropathy. There are two main types: **a primary arteriovenous fistula**, in which an artery and vein are anastomosed so that the vein subsequently dilates and arteriolizes, and the **arteriovenous graft**, in which an artificial graft is placed between the artery and the vein. Although the primary arteriovenous fistula may require up to 6 weeks to mature, it is preferred because the incidence of infection and thrombosis is greatly reduced. Unfortunately, a great many patients do not have the distal vasculature that can support a primary arteriovenous fistula. These include those patients with prior exposure to prolonged steroids, diabetics, intravenous drug users, and those with vasculitis. The arteriovenous graft can often be used within 1 to 2 weeks of placement or even in less time if necessary. The negatives to this alternative are related to the implantation of a foreign body in the form of the graft, thus increasing the risk of infection and thrombosis.

REFERENCES

1. Dahlberg PJ, Yutuc WR, Newcomer KL. Subclavian hemodialysis catheter infections. Am J Kidney Dis 1986;7:421–427.
2. Maki DG, Weise CE, Sarafin HWA. A semiquantitative culture method for identifying intravenous-catheter related infection. N Engl J Med 1977;296:1305–1309.
3. Raad I, Darouiche R, Dupuis J, et al. Central venous catheters coated with minocycline and rifampin for the prevention of catheter-related colonization and bloodstream infections. Ann Intern Med 1997;127:267–274.
4. Maki DG, Stolz SM, Wheeler S, Mermel LA. Prevention of central venous catheter-related bloodstream infection by the use of an antiseptic-impregnated catheter: a randomized, controlled study. Ann Intern Med 1997;127:257–266.
5. Schwab SJ, Buller GJ, McCann RL, Bollinger RR, Stickel DL. Prospective evaluation of a Dacron cuffed hemodialysis

catheter for prolonged use. Am J Kidney Dis 1988;11:166–169.

6. Hannah A, Buttimore AL. Thrombolysis of blocked hemodialysis catheters using recombinant tissue-type plasminogen activator. Nephron 1991;59:517–518.

7. Mokrzycki MH, Kaplan AA. Therapeutic plasma exchange complications and management. Am J Kidney Dis 1994; 23:817–827.

8. Kjellstrand CM, Merino GE, Mauer SM, Casail R, Buselmeier TJ. Complications of percutaneous femoral vein catheterisation for hemodialysis. Clin Nephrol 1975;4:37–40.

9. Mansfield PF, Hohn DC, Fornage BD, Gregurich MA, Ota DM. Complications and failures of subclavian-vein catheterization. N Engl J Med 1994;331:1735–1738.

10. Haire WD, Lieberman RP. Defining the risks of subclavian-vein catheterization. N Engl J Med 1994;331:1769–1770. Editorial.

11. Spinowitz BS, Galler M, Golden RA, et al. Subclavian vein stenosis as a complication of subclavian catheterisation for hemodialysis. Arch Intern Med 1987;147:305–307.

12. Cimochowski GE, Worley E, Rutherford WE, Sartain J, Blondin J, Harter H. Superiority of the internal jugular over the subclavian access for temporary dialysis. Nephron 1990;54: 154–161.

13. Timsit JF, Sebille V, Farkas JC, Misset B, Martin JB, Chevret S, Carlet J. Effect of subcutaneous tunneling on internal jugular catheter-related sepsis in critically ill patients. A prospective randomized multicenter trial. JAMA 1996;276:1416–1420.

14. Fan P-Y, Schwab SJ. Vascular access: concepts for the 1990s. J Am Soc Nephrol 1992;3:1–11.

GENERAL REFERENCE

1. Udall R. Vascular access for continuous renal replacement therapy. Semin Dial 1996;9:93–97.

SELECTIVE PLASMAPHERESIS TECHNIQUES

Many imaginative techniques have been designed to selectively adsorb a particular pathogenic substance from the plasma, allowing most of the plasma to be returned to the patient, thus minimizing the risks of depletion coagulopathy and hypogammaglobulinemia (1,2). Although many of these systems are currently in use in Europe and Japan, only a few have been approved for use in the United States.

REFERENCES

1. Malchesky PS, Kaplan AA, Coo AP, Sadurada Y, Siami GA. Are selective macromolecule removal plasmapheresis systems useful for autoimmune diseases or hyperlipidemia? ASAIO J 1993;39: 868–872.
2. Samtleben W, Schmidt B, Gurland HJ. Ex vivo and in vivo protein A perfusion: background, basic investigations, and first clinical experiences. Blood Purif 1987;5:179–192.

Cascade Filtration ("Double Filtration")

Cascade filtration, or double filtration, plasmapheresis is a selective method of plasma fractionation in which the whole plasma separated from the cellular components is refiltered through a secondary filter with a smaller pore size to separate out the larger unwanted molecules (1,2). This type of selective removal limits the amount of replacement fluid that is required by allowing most of the smaller molecules like albumin (60,000 Da) to return to the patient. This methodology has been used to selectively remove the relatively large beta-lipoproteins (~1 million Da), IgM (900,000 Da), cryoglobulins, and immune complexes. In general, after a 1-liter exchange, approximately 60% of the albumin and 50% of the IgG (160,000 Da) are returned to the patient, whereas only 10 to 15% of the IgM or cholesterol-containing beta-lipoprotein is allowed to return (3). Although this technique is elegantly simple and has the clear advantage of limiting the risks of replacement fluid infusions and plasma component depletion, the separation of molecular components is not perfect and not without its "depletion" syndromes. In one report, a patient with cirrhosis-related cryoglobulinemia developed edema secondary to the inability of the liver to replenish even the modest albumin losses of this technique (4). Similarly, fibrinogen removal can lead to "depletion" coagulopathy. The secondary filters, with their smaller than normal filtration pores, have a tendency to clot, a situation that can be anticipated when the transmembrane pressure increases above 250 mm Hg. In a series of treatments involving approximately 3 liters of processed plasma, between two and six "rinse-back" procedures were required (4). Using a slightly larger pore-sized filter during initial treatments (0.1 versus 0.06 μm) may limit the tendency for filter clotting, as does raising the temperature of the filtration system to 42°C.

Cascade filtration has been used successfully for Waldenström's macroglobulinemia, cryoglobulinemia, familial hypercholesterolemia, and immune complex–mediated disease (4,5). Nonetheless, this technique must be evaluated in the context of the increased costs of the secondary filter, the increased duration and reduced efficiency of the treatments, and the general tendency of the secondary filters to clot. In one trial with double filtration, we were able to remove 4.9 g of cholesterol-containing lipoprotein with return of 80% of the processed plasma. Unfortunately, compared with standard TPE, this procedure required more time and removed significantly less cholesterol (4.9 versus 6.7 g) (6). Aside from these technical considerations, the secondary filters necessary for this type of circuit are increasingly difficult to find in the United States.

REFERENCES

1. Agishi T, Kaneko I, Hasuo Y, Hayasaka Y, Sanaka T, Ota K, Abe M, Ono T, Kawai S, Yamane K. Double filtration plasmapheresis. Trans Am Soc Artif Intern Organs 1980;26:406–409.
2. Sawada K, Malchesky PS, Nose Y. Available removal systems: state of the art. In: Nydegger UE, ed. Therapeutic hemapheresis in the 1990s. Current Studies in Hematology and Blood Transfusion. Basel: Karger, 1990:51–113.
3. Gurland HJ, Lysaght MJ, Samtleben W, Schmidt G. Comparative evaluation of filters used in membrane plasmapheresis. Nephron 1984;36:173–182.
4. Valbonisi M, Guzzini F, Servi D, Villa P, Montani F, Angelini G. Cascade filtration with reverse rinse of the secondary filter. J Clin Apheresis 1987;3:240–243.
5. Valbonesi M, Garelli S, Montani F, et al. Management of immune-mediated and paraproteinemic diseases by membrane plasma separation and cascade filtration. Vox Sang 1982;43: 91–101.
6. Kaplan AA, Halley SE, Reardon J, Sevigny J. One year's experience using a rotating filter for therapeutic plasma exchange. Trans Am Soc Artif Intern Organs 1989;35:262–264.

Cryofiltration

Cryofiltration is a technique in which the removed plasma is subjected to cooling by which certain pathogenic substances will aggregate, thus increasing their overall size and allowing efficient secondary filtration (1,2). The process can be used to selectively remove cryoglobulins and immune complexes. The technique is most efficiently performed by a continuous, online process requiring a specialized machine designed for this purpose (Cryomax, Parker Biomedical, Irvine, CA). Alternatively, one can perform a two-step procedure where the patient's own plasma can be reinfused after incubation in the cold to precipitate out the abnormal proteins (3).

REFERENCES

1. Vibert GJ, Wirtz SA, Smith JW, et al. Cryofiltration as an alternative to plasma exchange: plasma macromolecular solute removal without replacement fluids. In: Nose Y, Malchesky PS, Smith JW, eds. Plasmapheresis. Cleveland: ISAO Press, 1983: 281–287.
2. Sawada K, Malchesky PS, Nose Y. Available removal systems: state of the art. In: Nydegger UE, ed. Therapeutic hemapheresis in the 1990s. Current Studies in Hematology and Blood Transfusion. Basel: Karger, 1990:51–113.
3. McLeod BC, Sassetti RJ. Plasmapheresis with return of cryoglobulin-depleted autologous plasma (cryoglobulinpheresis) in cryoglobulinemia. Blood 1980;55:866–870.

Immunoadsorbant Techniques

There are several commercially available systems for selective immunoadsorption of a variety of targets. These systems may be designed for nonselective adsorption of immunoglobulins, such as those using protein A, or for more selective targets, such as those for the specific immunoadsorption of low-density-lipoprotein (LDL) cholesterol.

Protein A columns: Protein A is a 42,000-Da protein released from certain strains of *Staphylococcus aureus* and has been used for years in laboratories for the adsorption and purification of IgG. The protein can be attached to sepharose, collodion charcoal, or silica and can be used for the ex vivo adsorption of three of the four

Table 3-3. Protein A Immunoadsorption: Current and Potential Indications

Disease	Device	Reference
Idiopathic thrombocytopenic purpura (FDA approved)	Prosorba	Guthrie and Oral. Semin Hematol, 1989
Cancer-associated hemolytic uremic system	Prosorba	Korec et al. J Clin Oncol, 1986
Cancer	Prosorba	Messerschmidt et al. Semin Hematol, 1989
Thrombotic thrombocytopenic purpura	Prosorba	Mittleman et al. N Engl J Med, 1992
Transfusion refractory thrombocytopenia	Prosorba	Christrie et al. Transfusion, 1993
Anti-HLA antibodies in renal transplant candidates	Excorim	Hakim et al. Am J Kidney Dis, 1990
		Ross et al. Transplantation, 1993
Rapidly progressive glomerulonephritis	Excorim	Palmer et al. Nephrol Dial Transplant, 1991

classes of IgG (1, 2, and 4). Binding occurs at a particular site on the heavy chain of the immunoglobulin, leaving binding sites for complement and antigens unaffected (1). There are two systems currently used in clinical practice: the Prosorba column (Cypress Biosciences, San Diego, CA), which has been in use in the United States for several years, and the Excorim system, which is currently under Food and Drug Administration (FDA) review. Current and potential indications for these devices are listed in Table 3-3.

REFERENCE

1. Samtleben W, Schmidt B, Gurland HJ. Ex vivo and in vivo protein A perfusion: background, basic investigations and first clinical experience. Blood Purif 1987;5:179–192.

IMRE Prosorba column: The Prosorba column is a single-use non-regenerating system that is placed in series with a standard plasma exchange circuit. Once the plasma is separated from the blood, it is slowly perfused over the column (at 20 mL/min) where three of the four classes of IgG antibodies are selectively adsorbed onto the immobilized protein A. The treated plasma is then reinfused into the patient. The net amount of IgG removed is minimal when compared with a standard plasma exchange (1 versus 20 to 30 g) and the device is reported to work by some form of "immunomodulation." Possible modes of action include a particular propensity to remove immune complexes, the stimulation of anti-idiotypic antibodies, or the infusion of anaphylatoxin-producing substances, such as activated complement (1).

The Prosorba column is FDA approved for idiopathic thrombocytopenic purpura (ITP). In one study, the column was used on 10 patients with treatment-resistant immune thrombocytopenic purpura; a complete remission was obtained in 1 patient, partial remission in 4, and no response in 5 (2). Similar results were obtained in a more recent study involving patients refractory to platelet transfusions because of antiplatelet antibodies (3). The column has also been evaluated for other indications. In an uncontrolled trial, the column was used on 101 patients who had failed conventional antitumor therapy and in whom no antitumor medication was given for at least 4 weeks. Of these, there was a partial or less than partial response in 22%. Those with Kaposi's sarcoma and those with breast adenocarcinoma had the best response (4). In data obtained from a retrospective questionnaire, plasma perfusion over the Prosorba protein A column was reported to result in a successful treatment for 25 of 55 patients with chemotherapy-associated HUS/TTP (5). There is also an intriguing case report of its beneficial use in TTP (6). There is an ongoing FDA approval study for its use in breast cancer.

Secondary effects during the procedure are common and might be construed as evidence of the treatment's immunomodulation. In one large series involving 142 patients and 1306 treatments, 79% of patients experienced at least one episode of toxicity during the procedure, although 60% of treatments were free of side effects (7). The most common side effects were fever, chills, and musculoskeletal pains, but more severe reactions, such as hypotension, were also noted. These secondary effects may result from the release of activated complement products and seem to be the basis for the recommendation that plasma perfused over the device should not be reinfused into the patient at a rate exceeding 20 mL/min. For similar reasons, **the device should not be used in patients who are currently taking ACE inhibitors**, because these drugs block the degradation of bradykinins and may result in a severe anaphylactoid reaction as treated plasma is reinfused into the patient (8). A recent report suggests that this treatment was the cause of a systemic vasculitis (9).

REFERENCES

1. Snyder HW Jr, Balint JP, Jones FR. Modulation of immunity in patients with autoimmune disease and cancer treated by extra-corporeal immunoadsorption with Prosorba columns. Semin Hematol 1989;26:31–41.
2. Guthrie TH Jr, Oral A. Immune thrombocytopenia purpura: a pilot study of staphylococcal protein A immunomodulation in refractory patients. Semin Hematol 1989;26:3–9.
3. Christie DJ, Howe RB, Lennon SS, Sauro SC. Treatment of refractoriness to platelet transfusion by column therapy. Transfusion 1993;33:234–242.
4. Messerschmidt GL, Henry H, Snyder HW Jr, Bertram J, Mittelman A, Ainsworth S, Fiore J, Viola MV, Louie J, Ambinder E, MacKintosh FR, Higby DJ, O'Brien P, Kiprov D, Hamberger M, Balint JP Jr, Fisher LD, Perkins W, Pinsky CM, Jones FR. Protein A immunotherapy in the treatment of cancer: an update. Semin Hematol 1989;26:19–24.
5. Snyder HJ, Mittleman A, Oral A, Messerschmidt GL, Henry DH, Korec S, Bertram JH, Guthrie TH, Ciavarella D, Wuest D, Perkins W, Balint JP, Cochran SK, Peugeot RL, Jones FR. Treatment of cancer chemotherapy-associated thrombotic thrombocytopenic purpura/hemolytic uremic syndrome by protein A immunoad-sorption of plasma. Cancer 1993;71:1882–1892.
6. Mittleman A, Puccio C, Ahmed T, et al. Response of refractory thrombotic thrombocytopenic purpura to extracorporeal im-munoadsorption. N Engl J Med 1992;326:711. Letter.
7. Snyder HW Jr, Henry DH, Messerschmidt GL, et al. Minimal toxicity during protein A immunoadsorption treatment of malignant disease: an outpatient therapy. J Clin Apheresis 1991;6:1–10.
8. Brecher ME, Owen Hg, Collins ML. Apheresis and ACE inhibitors. Transfusion 1993;33:963–964. Letter.
9. Case presentation. N Engl J Med 1994;331:792–799.

Excorim: In sharp contrast to the Prosorba column described above, the Excorim protein A system uses a circuit in which two columns are repeatedly regenerated to allow for a much more efficient IgG removal (1). This regenerating system, which may soon be available in the United States, has demonstrated promising results in removing anti–human leukocyte antigen antibodies from candidates for renal transplant (2,3) and for the treatment of proliferative glomerulonephritis (4).

REFERENCES

1. Gjorstrup P, Watt RM. Therapeutic protein A immunoadsorption. A review. Transfus Sci 1990;11:281–302.
2. Hakim RM, Milford E, Himmelfarb J, Wingard R, Lazarus JM, Watt RM. Extracorporeal removal of anti-HLA antibodies in transplant candidates. Am J Kidney Dis 1990;16:423–431.
3. Ross CN, Gaskin G, Gregor-Macgregor S, Patel AA, Davey NJ, Lechler RI, Williams G, Rees AJ, Pusey CD. Renal transplantation following immunoadsorption in highly sensitized recipients. Transplantation 1993;55:785–789.
4. Palmer A, Cairns T, Dische F, Gluck G, Gjorstrup P, Parsons V, Welsh K, Taube D. Treatment of rapidly progressive glomerulonephritis by extracorporeal immunoadsorption, prednisolone and cyclophosphamide. Nephrol Dial Transplant 1991;6:536–542.

Selective Lipid Removal

Although standard plasma exchange can successfully lower serum cholesterol levels (1) (see section on hypercholesterolemia in Chap. 9), recent interest has been centered on the development of selective lipid removal techniques that can limit the loss of nonlipid-containing plasma proteins and desirable high-density-lipoprotein cholesterol. Of these, three have undergone extensive clinical trials in the United States. One is an immunoadsorbant system in which plasma is perfused over sepharose beads coated with antibodies against LDL (2). Another is a dextran sulfate system by which negatively charged dextran molecules are covalently bound to the positively charged apoprotein B lipoproteins (3), and a third is known as the heparin-induced extracorporeal LDL precipitation (HELP) system and involves the extracorporeal precipitation of LDL by negatively charged heparin (4). Although conceptually different in their approaches, an evaluation of all three techniques found them to be equally biocompatible and equally efficacious in lowering LDL cholesterol (5). Two reports, however, have warned of anaphylactoid reactions in patients treated with the dextran sulfate–based system in whom there was concurrent treatment with ACE inhibitors (6,7). Semiselective systems using thermofiltration or double cascade filtration have also been proposed (8–10).

A multicenter controlled trial of the immunoadsorbant system demonstrated that homozygous and heterozygous patients with familial hypercholesterolemia refractory to diet and drug therapy had statistically significant decreases in cholesterol as a result of biweekly treatments for 6 weeks (2). Perhaps more important and impressive are the results from a computerized evaluated coronary angiographic study that provided evidence of atherosclerotic regression in patients treated with drugs and the dextran sulfate lipid removal system (11). In agreement with these results, the most recent reports continue to support the concept that aggressive lipid lowering with extracorporeal removal techniques can result in clinically important regression of both coronary and peripheral vascular disease (12–14).

At present, two of the above systems are currently available in the United States: the Liposorba (Kaneka, distributed in the U.S. by Cobe CBT, Lakewood, CO), using immunoadsorbant technology, and the HELP system (Braun Melsungen AG, Melsungen, Germany), using a precipitation technique. There is an estimated 5 to 10,000 severe heterozygous or homozygous patients in the United States who would qualify for this treatment (homozygous, 1/million; heterozygous, 1/500).

REFERENCES

1. Berger GM, Miller JL, Bonnici F, Joffe HS, Dubovsky DW. Continuous flow plasma exchange in the treatment of homozygous familial hypercholesterolemia. Am J Med 1978;65:243–251.
2. Saal SD, Parker TS, Gordon BR. Removal of low-density lipoproteins in patients by extracorporeal immunoadsorption. Am J Med 1986;80:583–589.
3. Gordon BR, Kelsey SF, Bilheimer DW, Brown DC, Dau PC, Gotto AM Jr, Illingworth DR, Jones PH, Leitman SF, Prihoda JS, et al. Treatment of refractory familial hypercholesterolemia by low density lipoprotein apheresis using an automated dextran sulfate cellulose adsorption system. Am J Cardiol 1992; 70:1010–1016.
4. Eisenhauer T, Armstrong VW, Schuff-Werner P, et al. Long term clinical experience with HELP-CoA-reductase inhibitors for

maximum treatment of coronary heart disease associated with severe hypercholesterolemia. Trans Am Soc Artif Intern Organs 1989;35:580–583.

5. Schaumann D, Olbricht CJ, Welp M, et al. Extracorporeal removal of LDL-cholesterol: prospective evaluation of effectivity, selectivity and biocompatibility. J Am Soc Nephrol 1992; 3:392. Abstract.

6. Olbricht CJ, Schauman D, Fisher D. Anaphylactoid reactions, LDL apheresis with dextran sulfate and ACE inhibitors. Lancet 1992;340:908–909.

7. Kroon AA, Mol MJTM, Stalenhoff APH. ACE inhibitors and LDL-apheresis with dextran sulfate adsorption. Lancet 1992;340:1476.

8. Takeyama Y, Malchesky PS, Cressman MD. Removal and recovery of cholesterol in thermofiltration. Int J Artif Organs 1988;11:201–208.

9. Busnach G, Cappelleri A, Vaccarino V, et al. Selective and semi-selective low-density lipoprotein apheresis in familial hypercholesterolemia. Blood Purif 1988;6:156–161.

10. Kaplan AA, Halley SE, Reardon J, Sevigny J. One year's experience using a rotating filter for therapeutic plasma exchange. Trans Am Soc Artif Intern Organs 1989;35:262–264.

11. Tatami R, Inoue N, Itoh H, et al. Regression of coronary atherosclerosis by combined LDL-apheresis and lipid-lowering drug therapy in patients with familial hypercholesterolemia: a multicenter study. Atherosclerosis 1992;95:1–13.

12. Kroon AA, van Asten WNJC, Stalenhoef AFH. Effect of apheresis of low-density lipoprotein on peripheral vascular disease in hypercholesterolemic patients with coronary artery disease. Ann Intern Med 1996;125:945–954.

13. Aengevaeren WR, Kroon AA, Stalenhoef AF, Uijen GJ, van der Werf T. Low density lipoprotein apheresis improves regional myocardial perfusion in patients with hypercholesterolemia and extensive coronary artery disease. LDL-Apheresis Atherosclerosis Regression Study (LAARS). J Am Coll Cardiol 1996;28:1696–1704.

14. Kroon AA, Aengevaeren WR, van der Werf T, Uijen GJ, Reiber JH, Bruschke AV, Stalenhoef AF. LDL-Apheresis Atherosclerosis Regression Study (LAARS). Effect of aggressive versus conventional lipid lowering treatment on coronary atherosclerosis. Circulation 1996;93:1826–1835.

Endotoxin Adsorption

The removal of endotoxin represents a promising role for extracorporeal blood purification techniques. In essence, the body has only limited means for the removal of these large-molecular-weight toxins that can include fragments of several hundred thousand daltons or more. Under conditions of sepsis, the reticuloendothelial system becomes overloaded and these toxic fragments are trapped in the circulation, stimulating a host of inflammatory processes by way of cytokines, eicosanoids, and nitric oxide. Although standard TPE can successfully remove circulating endotoxins (see Chap. 13), selective adsorption is particularly appealing because FFP will not be required, thus avoiding depleting the critically ill patient of immunoglobulins and clotting factors. Selective adsorption can be accomplished by filters impregnated with polymyxin B, an antibiotic that has the particular propensity to bind endotoxin fragments. Several publications from Japan documented the clinical application of this filter, demonstrating a concomitant improvement in systemic hemodynamics as endotoxin levels were lowered (1–3). Unfortunately, this device is not currently available in the United States.

REFERENCES

1. Hanasawa K, Aoki H, Yoshioka T, Matsuda K, Tani T, Kodama M. Novel mechanical assistance in the treatment of endotoxic and septicemic shock. Am Soc Artif Intern Organs Trans 1989;35:341–343.
2. Kodama M, Aoki H, Tani T, Hanasawa K. Hemoperfusion using a polymyxin B immobilized fiber column for the removal of endotoxin. In: Levin J, Alving CR, Munford RS, Stutz PL, eds. Bacterial endotoxin: recognition and effector mechanisms. Amsterdam: Elsevier Science Publishers B.V., 1993:389–398.
3. Aoki H, Kodama M, Tani T, Hanasawa K. Treatment of sepsis by extracorporeal elimination of endotoxin using polymyxin B-immobilized fiber. Am J Surg 1994;167:412–417.

Complications and Management

4

Citrate-Induced Hypocalcemia   56
Coagulation Abnormalities   59
  "Depletion" Coagulopathy   59
  Thrombocytopenia   60
  Anemia   60
  Thrombosis   62
Infection   63
  Postpheresis Infection   64
  Risk of Viral Transmission   65
Reactions to Protein-Containing Replacement Fluids   69
Atypical Reactions Associated with Angiotensin-Converting Enzyme Inhibitors   71
Electrolyte Abnormalities   72
  Hypokalemia   72
  Alkalosis   72
  Aluminum   72
Vitamin Removal   73
Miscellaneous Complications   74
Hypotension   75
Deaths   76

Although several reviews identified the potential risks of therapeutic plasmapheresis (1–3), only a few large series allowed the clinician to assess the incidence of these complications (4–12). Complications reported in these nine series, involving over 15,000 therapeutic plasma exchange (TPE) treatments, reveal that the most common complications are citrate-induced paresthesias, muscle cramps, and urticaria (Table 4-1) (12). More serious complications are reported at a rate of 0.025 to 0.2% and include life-threatening anaphylactoid reactions that are most commonly associated with the use of fresh frozen plasma (FFP) (13).

Table 4-1. Complications of Plasmapheresis

Symptom	Percentage
Urticaria	0.7–12
Paresthesias	1.5–9
Muscle cramps	0.4–2.5
Dizziness	<2.5
Headaches	0.3–5
Nausea	0.1–1
Hypotension	0.4–4.2
Chest pain	0.03–1.3
Dysrhythmia	0.1–0.7
Anaphylactoid reactions	0.03–0.7
Rigors	1.1–8.8
Hyperthermia	0.7–1.0
Bronchospasm	0.1–0.4
Seizure	0.03–0.4
Respiratory arrest/pulmonary edema	0.2–0.3
Myocardial ischemia	0.1
Shock/MI	0.1–1.5
Metabolic alkalosis	0.03
DIC	0.03
CNS ischemia	0.03–0.1
Hepatitis	0.7
Hemorrhage	0.2
Hypoxemia	0.1
Pulmonary embolism	0.1
Access related	
Thrombosis/hemorrhage	0.02–0.7
Infection	0.3
Pneumothorax	0.1
Mechanical	0.08–4

MI, myocardial infarction; DIC, disseminated intravascular coagulation; CNS, central nervous system.
SOURCE: Data are from references 4–12 comprising over 15,000 treatments. Adapted from Mokrzycki MH, Kaplan AA. Therapeutic plasma exchange: complications and management. Am J Kidney Dis 1994;23:817.

The overall incidence of death is 0.05%, but many of these report-edly "treatment-associated" deaths were in patients with severe pre-existing conditions in which TPE may not have been the precipitating cause.

REFERENCES

1. Isbister JP. The risk/benefit equation for therapeutic plasma exchange. In: Nydegger UE, ed. Therapeutic hemapheresis in the 1990s. Basel, Switzerland: Karger AG, 1990:10–30.
2. Hazards of apheresis. Lancet 1982;2:1025–1026. Editorial.
3. Westphal RG. Complications of hemapheresis. In: Westphal RG, Kasprisin DO, eds. Current status of hemapheresis: indications, technology and complications. Arlington, VA: American Association of Blood Banks, 1987:87–104.
4. Borberg H. Problems of plasma exchange therapy. In: Gurland HJ, Heinze V, Lee HA, eds. Therapeutic plasma exchange. New York: Springer-Verlag, 1980:191–201.
5. Aufeuvre JP, Morin-Hertel F, Cohen-Solal M, Lefloch A, Baudelot J. Hazards of plasma exchange. In: Sieberth HG, ed. Plasma exchange. Stuttgart, Germany: FK Schattauer Verlag, 1980:149–157.
6. Ziselman EM, Bongiovanni MB, Wurzel HA. The complications of therapeutic plasma exchange. Vox Sang 1984;46:270–276.
7. Fabre M, Andreu G, Mannoni P. Some biological modifications and clinical hazards observed during plasma exchanges. In: Seiberth HG, ed. Plasma exchange. Stuttgart, Germany: FK Schattauer Verlag, 1980:143–148.
8. Rossi PL, Cecchini L, Minichella G, De Rosa G, Alfano G, Pieralla L, Testa A, Candido A, Vittorio M, Mango G. Comparison of the side effects of therapeutic cytapheresis and those of other types of hemapheresis. Haematologica 1991;76(suppl 1):75–80.
9. Sprenger KBG, Rasche H, Franz HE. Membrane plasma separation: complications and monitoring. Artif Organs 1984;8:360–363.
10. Samtleben W, Hillebrand G, Krumme D, Gurland HJ. Membrane plasma separation: clinical experience with more than 120 plasma exchanges. In: Sieverth HG, ed. Plasma exchange. Stuttgart, Germany: FK Schattauer Verlag, 1980:23–27.
11. Sutton DMC, Nair RC, Rock G, the Canadian Apheresis Study Group. Complications of plasma exchange. Transfusion 1989;29:124–127.
12. Mokrzycki MH, Kaplan AA. Therapeutic plasma exchange: complications and management. Am J Kidney Dis 1994;23:817–827.

13. Flaum MA, Cuneo RA, Appelbaum FR, Disseroth AB, Engel WK, Gralnick HR. The hemostatic imbalance of plasma exchange transfusion. Blood 1979;54:694–702.

CITRATE-INDUCED HYPOCALCEMIA

Citrate, infused either as the treatment's anticoagulant or in the FFP administered as the replacement fluid, will complex calcium and result in symptoms of hypocalcemia. These symptoms represent one of the more common complications of TPE and are reported to occur in up to 9% of treatments (1). The incidence is highest in those treatments using FFP as the replacement fluid, because this preparation is approximately 15% citrate by volume. Most often, the patient will complain of perioral or distal extremity tingling or paresthesias. More ominous, however, are the reports that citrate-induced hypocalcemia may be associated with prolongation of the QT interval on electrocardiogram, thus potentially increasing the risk of cardiac arrhythmia (2,3).

Widely used protocols suggest that citrate toxicity can be reasonably well controlled with the oral administration of calcium tablets during the procedure, reserving intravenous calcium replacement only for those who develop symptoms. In contrast, the prophylactic replacement of intravenous calcium has been found to significantly reduce the incidence of citrate-induced paresthesias (1,4,5). Hester et al (2) recommended calcium replacement with 10 mL of 10% calcium gluconate infused over 15 minutes approximately halfway through the procedure, whereas the citrate infusion rate should be limited to between 1.0 and 1.8 mg/kg/min. Our own protocol involves the infusion of 0.7 mg/kg/min of citrate, with prophylactic calcium (10 mL of 10% calcium chloride solution) administered 15 minutes after the beginning of the treatment and infused over a 15- to 30-minute period (5). For prolonged treatments, an additional 10 mL of calcium is administered at the 1-hour point. Ilamathi et al (6) reported the use of regional citrate anticoagulation for membrane plasma separation, using 22 mL/hr of citrate solution neutralized with 15 mL/hr of 10% calcium chloride solution. Others recommended a more conservative approach that involves decreasing the rate of plasma exchange and decreasing the citrate:blood ratio and supplementing with heparin (7–9).

Although kinetic studies demonstrated that increases in parathyroid hormone provide an endogenous compensatory

Table 4-2. Calcium Kinetics with and without Supplemental Infusion

Patient	Total Calcium Serum		Discarded Plasma	Total Removed	Supplement[a]	Replacement Fluid#	Net Balance
	Pre-Rx	Post-Rx					
	mg/dL					*mg*	
No supplement							
2	8.6	7.1	7.4	235	—	87	−148
3	8.9	6.9	7.4	235	—	87	−148
3	9.5	8.2	7.6	242	—	87	−155
With supplement							
2	9.3	9.2	8.7	261	273	87	+99
3	9.4	9.0	8.8	280	273	87	+80

To convert mg/dL to mEq/L, divide by 1.95; to convert mg to mEq, divide by 19.5. All treatments involved 3-liter exchanges.

[a] 10-mL ampule of 10% $CaCl_2$.

[b] 5% albumin solution with measured calcium concentration of 2.9 mg/dL.

Rx, treatment.

SOURCE: Reproduced by permission from Kaplan AA, Halley SE. Plasma exchange with a rotating filter. Kidney Int 1990;38:160–166.

response to calcium removal during TPE (7), patients receiving multiple treatments for prolonged periods experience a significant loss of calcium, amounting to approximately 150 mg per treatment (Table 4-2) (5). In contrast, with supplementation, calcium balance is positive by 90 mg.

Most recently, Uhl et al (10) described a case of severe citrate toxicity when the citrate infusion line became disengaged from its rotary pump. Seven minutes into the procedure, the patient developed signs and symptoms suggesting severe hypocalcemia, including muscle spasms, chest pain, and hypotension. Ionized calcium level was 0.64 mmol/L (normal range, 1.18 to 1.38 mmol/L). Thus, life-threatening hypocalcemia can occur if the citrate anticoagulant line of an apheresis instrument is not properly housed in its rotary pump or becomes disengaged during the procedure.

REFERENCES

1. Mokrzycki MH, Kaplan AA. Therapeutic plasma exchange: complications and management. Am J Kidney Dis 1994;23: 817–827.
2. Hester JP, McCullough J, Mishler JM, Szymanski IO. Dosage regimens for citrate anticoagulants. J Clin Apheresis 1983;1: 149–157.
3. Olson PR, Cox C, McCullough J. Laboratory and clinical effects of the infusion of ACD solution during platelet-pheresis. Vox Sang 1977;33:79–87.
4. Buskard NA, Varghese Z, Wills MR. Correction of hypocalcemic symptoms during plasma exchange. Lancet 1976;2: 344–345.
5. Kaplan AA, Halley SE. Plasma exchange with a rotating filter. Kidney Int 1990;38:160–166.
6. Ilamathi E, Kirsch M, Moore B, Finger M. Citrate anticoagulation during plasmapheresis using standard hemodialysis equipment. Semin Dial 1993;6:268.
7. Sutton DMC, Nair RC, Rock G, the Canadian Apheresis Study Group. Complications of plasma exchange. Transfusion 1989;29:124–127.
8. Silberstein LE, Naryshkin S, Haddad JJ, Strauss JF. Calcium homeostasis during therapeutic plasma exchange. Transfusion 1986;26:151–155.
9. Huestis DW. Complications of therapeutic apheresis. In: Pinada

AA, Valbonesi M, Diggs JC, eds. Therapeutic hemapheresis. Milan, Italy: Wichtig Editore, 1986:179–186.
10. Uhl L, Maillet S, King S, Kruskall MS. Unexpected citrate toxicity and severe hypocalcemia during apheresis. Transfusion 1997;37:1063–1065.

COAGULATION ABNORMALITIES
"Depletion" Coagulopathy

When albumin is used as the replacement fluid, a depletion of all coagulation factors occurs, including fibrinogen and antithrombin III (AT-III) (1–3). **After a single plasma exchange**, the serum levels of most of these factors are decreased by approximately 60% (Table 4-3). Rebound of these decreased levels is biphasic, characterized by a rapid initial increase in the first 4 hours after treatment, followed by a slower increase over the next few days (1). This dual rate of recovery probably represents a relatively rapid initial re-equilibration of extravascular stores with the intravascular compartment, followed by a slower rate of resynthesis. Twenty-four hours after treatment, fibrinogen levels are 50% and AT-III levels are 85% of initial levels, whereas both factors may require 48 to 72 hours for complete recovery (1). Prothrombin time (PT) increases 30% and partial thromboplastin time (PTT) doubles immediately after treatment (4). PTT and thrombin time are back to normal range 4 hours postpheresis, whereas PT normalizes in 24 hours (3).

Table 4-3. Percent Decrease in Serum Levels of Coagulation Factors After a Single Plasma Exchange

	Percent Decrease
Fibrinogen	20
Prothrombin	40
Factor V	42
Factor VII	47
Factor VIII	50
Factor IX	57
Factor X	32
AT-III	42

SOURCE: Modified from Chrinside A, Urbarick SJ, Promse CV, Killer AJ. Coagulation abnormalities following intensive plasma exchange on the cell separator. Br J Haematol 1981;48:627–634.

When multiple treatments are performed over a short period (i.e., three or more treatments per week), the depletion in clotting factors is more pronounced and may require several days for spontaneous recovery (1,2,4). Under these conditions, the risks of hemorrhage can be minimized by substituting between 500 and 1000 mL (2 to 4 units) of FFP as the replacement fluid for the end of the procedure (Fig 4-1). This approach is most helpful in patients immediately after surgery (i.e., thymectomy for myasthenia gravis), who have had a recent renal biopsy (i.e., glomerulonephritis), who have active hemoptysis (Goodpasture's syndrome or Wegener's granulomatosis), or in whom there is a desire for the immediate removal of a large-bore intravascular catheter.

Thrombocytopenia

Decreases in platelet count depend on the method of treatment. Whereas the older centrifugal methods were associated with decreases of up to 50%, the newer centrifugal devices provide more efficient plasma separation and a more modest decrease. Membrane plasma separation can result in a 15% decrease in platelet count (3–6). Thrombocytopenia may result from a loss of platelets in the discarded plasma, as a result of thrombosis within the plasma filter, or as a result of a mild dilutional effect by the infusion of relatively hyperoncotic replacement fluid.

Anemia

Although relatively uncommon (7), post-treatment decreases in hematocrit may result from hemorrhage associated with vascular access (see Vascular Access, Chap. 3) or from treatment-related

Figure 4-1. Changes in PTT as a result of plasma exchange with 5% albumin. Solid lines connect pre- and post-treatment values. Dotted lines are provided to demonstrate continuity in time with respect to post-treatment values. (A) Note the rapid return toward normal within 5 hours' post-treatment despite two successive treatments. (B) Despite some correction toward normal during the intertreatment periods, there is a tendency toward increasing pre-treatment values of PTT as the depletion coagulopathy becomes more profound. Twenty-four hours after the fourth treatment, the PTT is still moderately elevated. (C) Post-treatment coagulopathy was blunted by the infusion of 1 liter of FFP as the last liter of replacement fluid during each 4-liter exchange.

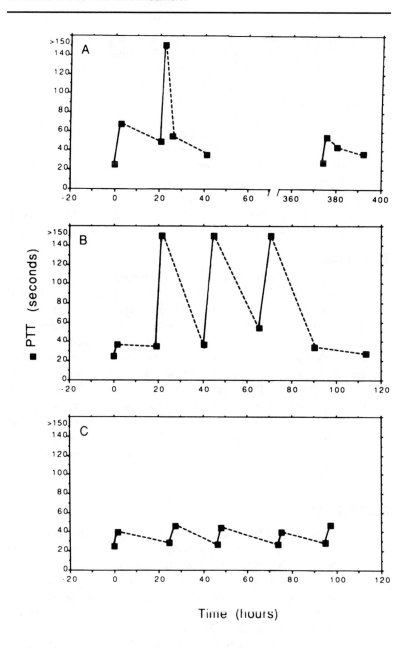

hemolysis. Initiation of treatment with a membrane plasma separa-tor is often associated with a minimal amount of plasma tinting that is rarely a cause for significant blood loss and can be quanti-fied by measuring the free hemoglobin levels in the collected plasma. In most cases, plasma tinting lasts for only a few seconds; if persistent, the blood flow should be slowed until the transmem-brane pressure can be evaluated (see TPE with Dialysis Equipment, Chap. 3). Hemolysis can also occur in centrifugal systems as a result of inappropriately hypotonic priming solution. Even in the absence of any extracorporeal losses or hemolysis, hematocrits may decrease by 10% after each treatment, a phenomenon that may be due to intravascular expansion related to the use of relatively hyperoncotic replacement solutions (4,8,9).

Thrombosis

As noted above, TPE treatments using albumin replacement cause a relative depletion of all coagulation factors, including AT-III and other inhibitors of coagulation. In one report, two episodes of thrombosis were associated with a postpheresis depletion of AT-III and the possibility that this deficiency may have resulted in a hyper-coaguable state (10). In our experience, rare cases of thrombosis have been associated with the prolonged use of indwelling vascu-lar catheters (7). Pulmonary embolism, cerebral ischemia, and myocardial infarction have been reported to occur in association with TPE, but the incidence is rare (0.06 to 0.14%) (11,12). An association with low levels of AT-III is speculative, especially because these patients also have a concomitant depletion of "pro"-coagulant factors (see above).

REFERENCES

1. Chrinside A, Urbaniak SJ, Prowse CV, Keller AJ. Coagulation abnormalities following intensive plasma exchange on the cell separator. Br J Haematol 1981;48:627–634.
2. Gelabert A, Puig L, Maragall S, Monteagudo J, Castillo R. Coagulation alterations during massive plasmapheresis. In: Sieverth HG, ed. Plasma exchange. Stuttgart, Germany: FK Schattauer Verlag, 1980:71–75.
3. Flaum MA, Cuneo RA, Appelbaum FR, Disseroth AB, Engel WK, Gralnick HR. The hemostatic imbalance of plasma exchange transfusion. Blood 1979;54:694–702.

4. Kaplan AA, Halley SE. Plasma exchange with a rotating filter. Kidney Int 1990;38:160–166.

5. Gurland HJ, Lysaght MJ, Samtleben W, Schmidt B. A comparison of centrifugal and membrane based apheresis formats. Int J Artif Organs 1984;7:35–38.

6. Keller AJ, Chirnside A, Urbaniak SJ. Coagulation abnormalities produced by plasma exchange on the cell separator with special reference to fibrinogen and platelet levels. Br J Haematol 1979;42:593–603.

7. Mokrzycki MH, Kaplan AA. Therapeutic plasma exchange: complications and management. Am J Kidney Dis 1994;23: 817–827.

8. Chopek M, McCullough J. Protein and biochemical changes during plasma exchange. In: Ulmas J, Berkman E, eds. Therapeutic hemapheresis: a technical workshop. Washington, DC: American Association of Blood Banks, 1980:13–52.

9. Wood L, Jacobs P. The effect of serial therapeutic plasmapheresis on platelet count, coagulation factors, plasma immunoglobulin and complement levels. J Clin Apheresis 1986;3:124–128.

10. Sultan Y, Bussel A, Maisonneuve P, Sitty X, Gajdos P. Potential danger of thrombosis after plasma exchange in the treatment of patients with immune disease. Transfusion 1979;19:588–593.

11. Aufeuvre JP, Mortin-Hertel F, Cohen-Solal M, Lefloch A, Baudelot J. Clinical tolerance and hazards of plasma exchanges: a study of 6200 plasma exchanges in 1033 patients. In Beyer JH, Burgerg H, Fuchs C, Nagel GA, eds. Plasmapheresis in immunology and oncology. Basel, Switzerland: Karger, 1982:65–77.

12. Ziselman EM, Bongiovanni MB, Wurzel HA. The complications of therapeutic plasma exchange. Vox Sang 1984;46: 270–276.

INFECTION

The risk of infection associated with TPE can be divided into two broad categories: those that may be the result of a post-treatment depletion of immunoglobulins, a situation most likely to occur when the replacement fluid is mostly albumin, and those that occur as a result of viral transmission from the replacement fluid, most likely to occur with FFP.

Postpheresis Infection

When albumin is used as the replacement fluid, removal of immunoglobulins and complement may predispose patients to high rates of infection. One plasma volume exchange results in a 60% reduction in serum immunoglobulin levels and a net 20% reduction in total body immunoglobulin stores (see Kinetics of Immunoglobulin Removal, Chap. 2) (1–3). Multiple treatments over short periods, especially when associated with immunosuppressive agents, yield a substantial decrease in immunoglobulin levels that may persist for several weeks (4–6). Although concentrations of C3 and C4 may be depleted by a series of daily treatments, because of their rather short half-lives, levels of these proteins rebound within several days. CH_{50} can be predictably lowered to about 40% of its initial value immediately after a given treatment, but rebound to pretreatment values occurs within 1 day, and even repetitive daily treatments have a minimal effect on this parameter, possibly because of its dependency on multiple factors (5). TPE with FFP replacement would not be expected to deplete immunoglobulin or complement levels.

The incidence of infection in patients undergoing TPE varies widely, and its pathogenesis is a matter of controversy. Wing et al (7) compared the incidence of infection in patients with rapidly progressive glomerulonephritis (RPGN) who received standard therapy (steroids and cytotoxic agents) with or without plasma exchange. A significantly high occurrence of opportunistic infections was found among the apheresis–treated group. Nonetheless, some of the control subjects were taken from retrospective review and granulocytopenia was present in two of five TPE-treated patients who developed infections, a condition that was more likely to be the result of the cytotoxic therapy than from the plasma exchange procedure per se. In other studies of RPGN, nine episodes of infection were found in 34 patients treated with TPE and immunosuppression, four resulting in death (8–16). Two of these nine patients were granulocytopenic (8,14). Data from patients with myasthenia gravis suggest a lower incidence of infection than in patients with renal disease (17–21). Thirty-six patients with myasthenia gravis received plasma exchange in addition to prednisone and azathioprine and were followed for a mean period of 9 months. Of these, only one patient developed an infectious complication (19).

In the only prospective randomized trial to address this issue, Pohl et al (20) studied 86 patients with lupus nephritis receiving cyclophosphamide and steroids with or without TPE. These investigators found no increase in the rate of infection or in infection-related deaths in the apheresis-treated group. In patients treated with TPE, the infection rate was 1.22 infections per 200 weeks with three deaths, compared with 1.15 infections per 200 weeks and four deaths in the control group. Thus, in the only prospective study in which the effect of TPE could be isolated from that of drug-induced immunosuppression, treatment with TPE was not associated with any increased risk of infection.

The above results do not rule out the possibility that immunoglobulin or complement depletion may impair a patient's ability to combat an ongoing infection. Thus, if a severe infection develops in the immediate postpheresis period, a reasonable approach would be to reconstitute normal immunoglobulin levels with a single infusion of intravenous immunoglobulin (IVIG) (100–400 mg/kg intravenously) (23), similar to the replacement dose recommended in patients with hypo- or agammaglobulinemia (24,25). Because of the relatively long half-life of IgG (21 days), this approach provides normalized immunoglobulin levels for several weeks, provided there are no further TPE treatments.

Risk of Viral Transmission

Risk of viral transmission during plasma exchange is directly related to replacement with FFP. Albumin preparations are treated with heat and are considered to be devoid of transmissible virus (26). The same claims were made for IVIGs, but an outbreak of hepatitis C from contaminated IVIG has been documented (27) and new methodologies for avoiding viral transmission from IVIG preparations have been initiated (28). In a review of listed complications from over 15,000 treatments, there was only one reported case of latent non-A/non-B hepatitis infection (29). Transmission of the human immunodeficiency virus (HIV) through therapeutic plasmapheresis is unlikely and would be anticipated as the result of infected FFP (30). The current incidence of transfusion-acquired viral infections has declined substantially from the early 1980s and is currently estimated as 1 in 63,000 units for hepatitis B, 1 in 100,000 units for hepatitis C, 1 in 680,000 units for HIV, and 1 in 641,000 units for human T-cell lymphotropic virus (31–33) (Table 4-4). It should be noted that FFP is normally provided in units of

Table 4-4.   Risk of Transfusion-Transmitted Viral Infections per Unit Transfused in the Mid-1990s

	Incidence
HIV	1/680,000
HCV	1/103,000
HTLV	1/641,000
HBV	1/63,000

Estimates are for the United States and assume the use of modern screening tests.
HCV, hepatitis C virus; HTLV, human T-cell lymphotropic virus; HBV, hapatitis B virus.
SOURCE: Combined data from references 31–33.

200 to 300 mL, such that a single plasma volume exchange with FFP (~3 liters) involves the infusion of 10 to 15 units obtained from an equal number of different donors.

REFERENCES

1. Kaplan AA, Halley SE. Plasma exchange with a rotating filter. Kidney Int 1990;38:160–166.
2. Keller AJ, Chirnside A, Urbaniak SJ. Coagulation abnormalities produced by plasma exchange on the cell separator with special reference to fibrinogen and platelet levels. Br J Haematol 1979;42:593–603.
3. Chopek M, McCullough J. Protein and biochemical changes during plasma exchange. In: Ulmas J, Berkman E, eds. Therapeutic hemapheresis: a technical workshop. Washington, DC: American Association of Blood Banks, 1980:13–52.
4. Sultan Y, Bussel A, Maisonneuve P, Sitty X, Gajdos P. Potential danger of thrombosis after plasma exchange in the treatment of patients with immune disease. Transfusion 1979;19:588–593.
5. Keller AJ, Urbaniak SJ. Intensive plasma exchange on the cell separator. Effects on serum immunoglobulins and complement components. Br J Haematol 1978;38:531–540.
6. Kaplan AA. Towards a rational prescription of plasma exchange: the kinetics of immunoglobulin removal. Semin Dial 1992;5: 227–229. Editorial.
7. Wing EJ, Bruns FJ, Fraley DS, Segel DP, Adler S. Infectious complications with plasmapheresis in rapidly progressive glomerulonephritis. JAMA 1980;244:2423–2426.

8. Lockwood CM, Pinching AJ, Sweny PM, Rees AJ, Pussell B, Uff J, Peters DK. Plasma exchange and immunosuppression in the treatment of fulminating immune-complex crescentic nephritis. Lancet 1977;1:63–67.

9. Rossen RD, Hersh EM, Sharp JT, McCredie KB, Gyorkey F, Suki WN, Eknoyan G, Reisberg MA. Effect of plasma exchange on circulating immune complexes and antibody formation in patients treated with cyclophosphamide and prednisone. Am J Med 1977;63:674–682.

10. Lockwood CM, Pearson TA, Rees AJ, Evans DJ, Peters DK, Wilson CB. Immunosuppression and plasma-exchange in the treatment of Goodpasture's syndrome. Lancet 1976;1:711–715.

11. Johnson JP, Whitman W, Briggs WA, Wilson CB. Plasmapheresis and immunosuppressive agents in antibasement membrane antibody-induced Goodpasture's syndrome. Am J Med 1978;64:354–359.

12. Depner TA, Chafin ME, Wilson CB, Gulyassy PF. Plasmapheresis for severe Goodpasture's syndrome. Kidney Int 1976;8:409. Abstract.

13. Lang CH, Brown DC, Staley N, Johnson G, Ma KQ, Border WA, Dalmasso AP. Goodpasture's syndrome treated with immunosuppression and plasma exchange. Arch Intern Med 1977;137:1076–1078.

14. Rosenblatt SG, Knight W, Bannayan GA, Wilson CB, Stein JH. Treatment of Goodpasture's syndrome with plasmapheresis. Am J Med 1979;66:689–696.

15. Walker RG, Dapice AJF, Becker GJ, Kincaid-Smith P, Craswell PW. Plasmapheresis in Goodpasture's syndrome with renal failure. Med J Aust 1979;1:875–879.

16. McKenzie PE, Taylor AE, Woodroffe AJ, Seymour AE, Chan YL, Clarkson AR. Plasmapheresis in glomerulonephritis. Clin Nephrol 1979;12:97–108.

17. Pinching AJ, Peters DK, Davis JN. Remission of myasthenia gravis following plasma-exchange. Lancet 1976;2:1373–1376.

18. Dau PC, Lindstrom JM, Cassel CK, Denys EH, Shev EE, Spitler LE. Plasmapheresis and immunosuppressive drug therapy in myasthenia gravis. N Engl J Med 1977;297:1134–1140.

19. Behan PO, Shakir RA, Simpson JA, Burnett AK, Allan TL, Haase G. Plasma-exchange combined with immunosuppressive therapy in myasthenia gravis. Lancet 1979;2:438–440.

20. Newsom-Davis J, Wilson SG, Vincent A, Ward CD. Long-term effects of repeated plasma exchange in myasthenia gravis. Lancet 1979;1:464–468.

21. Winklestein A, Volkin RL, Starz TW, Maxwell NG, Spero JA. The effects of plasma exchange on immunologic factors. Clin Res 1979;27:691. Abstract.

22. Pohl MA, Lan SP, Berl T, the Lupus Nephritis Collaborative Study Group. Plasmapheresis does not increase the risk for infection in immunosuppressed patients with severe lupus nephritis. Ann Intern Med 1991;114:924–929.

23. Mokrzycki MH, Kaplan AA. Therapeutic plasma exchange: complications and management. Am J Kidney Dis 1994;23: 817–827.

24. Consensus on IVIG. Lancet 1990;1:470–472.

25. Haas A. Use of intravenous immunoglobulin in immunoregulatory disorders. In: Stiehm ER, moderator. Intravenous immunoglobulins as therapeutic agents. Ann Intern Med 1987;107:367–382.

26. Finlayson JS. Albumin products. Semin Thromb Hemost 1980; 6:85–120.

27. Bjoro K, Froland SS, Yun Z, Samdal HH, Haaland T. Hepatitis C infection in patients with primary hypogammaglobulinemia after treatment with contaminated immune globulin. N Engl J Med 1994;331:1607–1611.

28. Schiff RI. Transmission of viral infections through intravenous immune globulin. N Eng J Med 1994;331:1649–1650. Editorial.

29. Fabre M, Andreu G, Mannoni P. Some biological modifications and clinical hazards observed during plasma exchanges. In: Seiberth HG, ed. Plasma exchange. Stuttgart, Germany: FK Schattauer Verlag, 1980:143–148.

30. Kiprov D, Simpson D, Romanick-Schmiedl S, Lippert R, Spira T, Busch D. Risk of AIDS-related virus (human immunodeficiency virus) transmission through apheresis procedures. J Clin Apheresis 1987;3:143–146.

31. Lackritz EM, Satten GA, Aberle-Grasse J, Dodd RY, Raimondi VP, Janssen RS, et al. Estimated risk of transmission of the human immunodeficiency virus by screened blood in the United States. N Eng J Med 1995;333:1721–1725.

32. Schreiber GB, Busch MP, Kleinman SH, Korelitz JJ. The risk of transfusion-transmitted virus invections. The Retrovirus Epidemiology Donor Study. N Engl J Med 1996;334:1685–1690.

33. AuBuchon JP, Birkmeyer JD, Busch MP. Safety of the blood supply in the United States: opportunities and controversies. Ann Intern Med 1997;127:904–909.

REACTIONS TO PROTEIN-CONTAINING REPLACEMENT FLUIDS (FFP, PLASMA PROTEIN FRACTION, ALBUMIN)

Reactions to FFP are anaphylactoid in nature and are characterized by fever, rigors, urticaria, wheezing, and hypotension and may eventually progress to laryngospasm (1,2). In a review of several large series, the reported incidence of this type of reaction was between 0.02 and 21% (3) (see Table 4-1). Although most reactions are limited to urticaria and rigors, the potential for life-threatening reactions is underscored by the list of 42 TPE-associated deaths compiled by Huestis (4), at least 30 of which were associated with FFP replacement. Similarly, Aufeuvre et al (5,6) reported seven deaths in 6200 treatments of which was noted non-hemodynamic pulmonary edema associated with FFP replacement. Sutton et al (7), in their review of over 5000 treatments from the Canadian Red Cross, reported eight patients with severe reactions comprised of severe urticaria, itching, shortness of breath, and wheezing and noted that all eight patients had been receiving plasma.

Human serum albumin consists of 96% albumin and trace amounts of alpha and beta globulins, and, as opposed to FFP, anaphylactoid reactions are rare and may be associated with the formation of antibodies to polymerized albumin created by heat treatment or stabilization with sodium caprylate (8,9). Recent reports suggested that patients taking angiotensin-converting enzyme (ACE) inhibitors may also be prone to an increased risk of "atypical" or hypotensive reactions to albumin (10,11).

There are several potential mechanisms that may trigger the anaphylactoid reactions described above: the presence of anti-IgA antibodies in a patient who is IgA deficient and who is receiving IgA-containing fluids (i.e., FFP, immunoglobulins); contamination of the replacement fluid with bacteria, endotoxins, or pyrogens; the presence of a prekallikrein activator and bradykinin, and the formation of antibodies to polymerized albumin (12).

Because of the relative high incidence of these reactions, patients undergoing massive replacement with FFP (i.e., for thrombotic thrombocytopenic purpura or hemolytic uremic syndrome) are commonly pretreated with 50 mg of diphenhydramine

(Benadryl; Parke-Davis). In those patients who have already demonstrated a sensitivity to FFP and in whom FFP replacement is obligatory (i.e., TTP), a successful prophylactic regimen has included 50 mg of prednisone given 13, 7, and 1 hour before the treatment; 50 mg of diphenhydramine given 1 hour before the treatment; and 25 mg of ephedrine given 1 hour before the treatment (12). **In the event of a severe life-threatening reaction (laryngeal edema, etc), 0.3–0.5 mL of epinephrine (1:1000 solution) should be available for subcutaneous administration.**

REFERENCES

1. Ring J, Messmer K. Incidence and severity of anaphylactoid reactions to colloid volume substitutes. Lancet 1977;1:466–469.
2. Bambauer R, Jutzler GA, Albrecht D, Keller HE, Kohler M. Indications of plasmapheresis and selection of different substitution solutions. Biomater Artif Cells Artif Organs 1989;17:9–27.
3. Mokrzycki MH, Kaplan AA. Therapeutic plasma exchange: complications and management. Am J Kidney Dis 1994;23:817–827.
4. Huestis DW. Mortality in therapeutic haemapheresis. Lancet 1983;1:1043. Letter.
5. Aufeuvre JP, Morin-Hertel F, Cohen-Solal M, Lefloch A, Baudelot J. Hazards of plasma exchange. In: Sieberth HG, ed. Plasma exchange. Stuttgart, Germany: FK Schattauer Verlag, 1980:149–157.
6. Aufeuvre JP, Mortin-Hertel F, Cohen-Solal M, Lefloch A, Baudelot J. Clinical tolerance and hazards of plasma exchanges: a study of 6200 plasma exchanges in 1033 patients. In: Beyer JH, Burgerg H, Fuchs C, Nagel GA, eds. Plasmapheresis in immunology and oncology. Basel, Switzerland: Karger, 1982:65–77.
7. Sutton DMC, Nair R, Rock G, the Canadian Apheresis Study Group. Complications of plasma exchange. Transfusion 1989;29:124–127.
8. Finlayson JS. Albumin products. Semin Thromb Hemost 1980;6:85–120.
9. Stafford CT, Lobel SA, Fruge BC, Moffitt JE, Hoff RG, Fadel HE. Anaphylaxis to human serum albumin. Ann Allergy 1988;61:85–88.

10. Brecher ME, Owen Hg, Collins ML. Apheresis and ACE inhibitors. Transfusion 1993;33:963–964.
11. Owen HG, Brecher ME. Atypical reactions associated with use of angiotensin-converting enzyme inhibitors and apheresis. Transfusion 1994;34:891–894.
12. Apter AJ, Kaplan AA. An approach to immunologic reactions with plasma exchange. J Allergy Clin Immunol 1992;90: 119–124.

ATYPICAL REACTIONS ASSOCIATED WITH ANGIOTENSIN-CONVERTING ENZYME INHIBITORS

ACE inhibitors are known to block the degradation of bradykinins and may result in severe anaphylactoid reactions if a given apheresis procedure results in the activation of kinins. Flushing, hypotension, abdominal cramping, and occasionally severe anaphylactoid reactions have been reported with the use of the dextran sulfate systems for selective lipid removal (1,2) and in patients treated with the Prosorba column (2). More recently, and rather disturbing, is a report describing atypical reactions in those patients receiving albumin replacement during standard apheresis (3). In one large review, all 14 patients (100%) who were receiving ACE inhibitor therapy during apheresis procedures experienced atypical reactions defined as flushing or hypotension (decrease of 20 mm Hg or more) (4). In contrast, only 20 (7%) of 285 patients not receiving ACE inhibitors developed atypical reactions ($p < 0.001$). The authors concluded that ACE inhibitors should be withheld for at least 24 hours before apheresis.

REFERENCES

1. Olbricht CJ, Schauman D, Fisher D. Anaphylactoid reactions, LDL apheresis with dextran sulphate and ACE inhibitors. Lancet 1992;340:908–909.
2. Kroon AA, Mol MJTM, Stalenhoff APH. ACE inhibitors and LDL-apheresis with dextran sulphate adsorption. Lancet 1992;340:1476.
3. Brecher ME, Owen Hg, Collins ML. Apheresis and ACE inhibitors. Transfusion 1993;33:963–964. Letter.
4. Owen HG, Brecher ME. Atypical reactions associated with use of angiotensin-converting enzyme inhibitors and apheresis. Transfusion 1994;34:891–894.

ELECTROLYTE ABNORMALITIES
Hypokalemia

Commercially available solutions of 5% albumin are isosmotic to plasma with a sodium level of approximately 145 mmol/L and a potassium level lower than 2 mmol/L (1). Thus, when albumin is used as the replacement fluid, a 25% reduction in serum potassium levels may occur in the immediate postpheresis period (2). With the most modern techniques, plasma exchange may be very rapid (2 to 3 L/hr) and there is the potential for hypokalemic arrhythmias during apheresis and in the immediate postpheresis period. Experience with dialysis–associated arrhythmias suggests that this type of hypokalemic arrhythmia is most likely to occur in the presence of digoxin and when potassium levels approach 2 mEq/L (3). Considering the above, we follow a protocol by which we add 4 mmol of potassium to each liter of 5% albumin.

Alkalosis

Metabolic alkalosis can result from large amounts of infused citrate. Formula B citrate solution is relatively isosmotic to plasma and contains 73 mmol/L of citrate, which, when metabolized, yields 219 mmol/L of bicarbonate. Formula A citrate solution is a hyperosmotic solution containing 252 mmol/L of sodium, and its 112 mmol/L of citrate yields 336 mmol/L of bicarbonate (see Table 3-2). FFP contains approximately 14% citrate solution by volume. In most patients, postpheresis bicarbonate levels are unchanged (2). In patients with renal failure, severe alkalemia may result from repeated treatments, especially when FFP is used as the replacement (4). In the most difficult circumstance, a patient with hemolytic uremic syndrome may require massive amounts of FFP while suffering from severe renal failure. In this case, alkalemia may become severe and frequent dialysis may be required to remove the excess bicarbonate. In this regard, if TPE and hemodialysis are required on the same day, it is preferable to perform the TPE first to allow the dialysis treatment to correct the citrate-induced alkalemia.

Aluminum

All albumin solutions are contaminated with between 4 and 24 mmol/L of aluminum (5,6). Repetitive plasma exchange with albumin may result in significant accumulation of aluminum. This is most likely to occur in patients with severe renal insufficiency, in whom 60 to 70% of infused aluminum is retained (6). Nonetheless, bone deposition of aluminum has been reported in a patient with normal renal function (5,6).

REFERENCES

1. Finlayson JS. Albumin products. Semin Thromb Hemost 1980;6:85–120.
2. Orlin JB, Berkman EM. Partial plasma exchange using albumin replacement: removal and recovery of normal plasma constituents. Blood 1980;56:1055–1059.
3. Morrison G, Michelson EL, Brown S, Morganroth J. Mechanism and prevention of cardiac arrhythmias in chronic hemodialysis patients. Kidney Int 1980;17:811–819.
4. Pearl RG, Rosenthal MH. Metabolic alkalosis due to plasmapheresis. Am J Med 1985;79:391–393.
5. Mousson C, Charhon SA, Ammar M, Accominotti M, Rifle G. Aluminum bone deposits in normal renal function patients after long-term treatment by plasma exchange. Int J Artif Organs 1989;23:664–667.
6. Milliner DS, Shinaberger JH, Shurman P, Coburn JW. Inadvertent aluminum administration during plasma exchange due to aluminum contamination of albumin replacement solutions. N Engl J Med 1985;312:165–167.

VITAMIN REMOVAL

After a single plasma exchange treatment, blood concentrations of vitamins B_{12}, B_6, A, C, and E and beta-carotene have been noted to decline between 24 and 48%, but there is a rebound to pretreatment levels within 24 hours (1). Possibly because of their large volumes of distribution as water-soluble vitamins, folate, thiamin, nicotinate, biotin, riboflavin, and pantothenate are not significantly altered by plasma exchange. The long-term effects of repetitive treatments are not known, but net removal of the protein-bound vitamin B_{12} is approximately 900 µg per treatment (2), and there is the potential for a substantial reduction in total body stores after repetitive treatments.

REFERENCES

1. Reddi A, Frank O, DeAngelis B, Jain R, Bashruddin I, Lasker N, Baker H. Vitamin status in patients undergoing single or multiple plasmapheresis. J Am Coll Nutr 1987;6:485–489.

2. Kaplan AA, Halley SE. Plasma exchange with a rotating filter. Kidney Int 1990;38:160–166.

MISCELLANEOUS COMPLICATIONS

Apneic events have been reported after plasma exchange in patients who had been anesthetized with succinylcholine (1,2). Succinylcholine is an anesthetic agent that is metabolized by cholinesterase, and these apneic events were considered to be the result of abnormally low post-treatment levels of plasma cholinesterase. Cholinesterase levels are reduced by 50% immediately after a single treatment (3). Levels less than 30% normal ($\sim$1000 U/L) are likely to be associated with decreased metabolism of succinylcholine (4,5). Because FFP contains normal levels of cholinesterase, depletion of this enzyme is only expected when albumin or plasma protein fraction (PPF) is used as replacement. Anesthetic agents dependent on serum cholinesterase for their metabolism should be used with caution immediately after plasma exchange, especially after a series of daily treatments. Repletion of cholinesterase with FFP may be a reasonable approach for treatments in the immediate perioperative period.

Adverse reactions (hypotension, dyspnea, and chest pain) may occur secondary to complement-mediated membrane bioincompatibility, similar to those described during hemodialysis (6). Anaphylactoid symptoms may also occur due to ethylene oxide sensitivity, which is used as a sterilizing agent (7). The incidence of filter-related leukocytopenia, thrombocytopenia, and hypocomplementemia is reduced with more biocompatible membranes, and reactions to ethylene oxide can be avoided with adequate priming of the filter (8). As previously noted, atypical reactions with flushing and hypotension have been described when TPE is performed in patients on ACE inhibitors (see Atypical Reactions Associated with ACE Inhibitors, above). Severe hemolysis occurs as a result of inappropriately hypotonic priming solutions and may result from overly aggressive transmembrane pressure during membrane plasma separation. Chills and other symptoms of hypothermia may be experienced because of inadequately warmed replacement fluid and can be avoided by warming the replacement solutions to body temperature.

REFERENCES

1. Keller AJ, Urbaniak SJ. Intensive plasma exchange on the cell separator. Effects on serum immunoglobulins and complement components. Br J Haematol 1978;38:531–540.
2. MacDonald R, Robinson A. Suxamethonium apnea associated with plasmapheresis. Anaesthesia 1980;35:198–201.
3. Wood GJ, Hall GM. Plasmapheresis and plasma cholinesterase. Br J Anaesth 1978;50:945–948.
4. Bowen RA. Anaesthesia in operations for the relief of hypertension. Anaesthesia 1960;15:3–10.
5. McCaul K, Robinson GD. Suxamethonium extension by tetrahydroaminoacrine. Br J Anaesth 1962;34:536–542.
6. Jorstad S. Biocompatibility of different hemodialysis and plasmapheresis membranes. Blood Purif 1987;5:123–137.
7. Nicholls AJ, Platts MM. Anaphylactoid reactions due to haemodialysis, haemofiltration or membrane plasma separation. BMJ 1982;285:1607–1609.
8. Aeschbacher B, Haeverli A, Nydegger UE. Donor safety and plasma quality in automated plasmapheresis. Vox Sang 1989;57:104–111.

HYPOTENSION

In several large series, the reported incidence of hypotension was 1.7% (see Table 4-1). Hypotension during TPE may occur for a variety of reasons, including delayed or inadequate volume replacement, vasovagal episodes, hypo-oncotic fluid replacement, anaphylaxis, cardiac arrhythmia, bradykinin reactions (cf. reactions to ACE inhibitors), vascular access–induced external or internal hemorrhage, and cardiovascular collapse (Table 4-5) (these issues are discussed in detail in the previous sections). Discontinuous-flow plasma exchange systems may be prone to a higher incidence of hypotensive episodes due to intermittent hypovolemia. The use of hypo-oncotic replacement solutions may also increase the risk of hypotensive events. In some institutions, albumin replacement fluid is prepared by dilution with an electrolyte solution to achieve a concentration of 3.5% albumin. In most patients, this solution is clearly hypo-oncotic to the patient's plasma and may predispose them to hypotension, even when a policy of 1:1 volume replacement is rigorously followed. An undiluted 5% albumin solution is

Table 4-5.   Potential Causes for Hypotension During TPE

Delayed or inadequate volume replacement
Vasovagal episodes
Hypo-oncotic fluid replacement
   3.5% albumin solutions
Anaphylaxis
   Reactions to plasma components in replacement fluids
   Anti-IgA antibodies (IgA-deficient patient)
   Endotoxin-contaminated replacement fluid
   Reactions to bioincompatible membranes
   Sensitivity to ethylene oxide
   Device related: Prosorba protein A column
Cardiac arrhythmia
   Citrate-induced hypocalcemia
   Hypokalemic related (especially in patients on digitalis)
Bradykinin reactions (cf. reactions to ACE inhibitors)
Hemorrhage
   Associated with primary disease (ITP, factor VIII inhibitors)
   Associated with heparin anticoagulation
   Associated with vascular access
      External
      Internal
   "Depletion" coagulopathy
Cardiovascular collapse
Pulmonary embolus
Disease-related hypotension
   Guillain-Barré syndrome (autonomic dysfunction)
   Waldenström's macroglobulinemia (rapid decrease in plasma volume)

See text for detailed discussion.
ITP, immune thrombocytopenic purpura.

less likely to produce a hypo-oncotic hypovolemia, except when pretreatment plasma volumes are abnormally expanded by a hyperviscosity state (Waldenström's macroglobulinemia).

DEATHS

In a review of the literature from 1983, Huestis (1) compiled a total of 42 deaths associated with therapeutic plasmapheresis, at least 30 of which were associated with FFP replacement. In five other cases, replacement solution was uncertain, and in the remaining six cases, albumin or PPF was used as replacement. The major causes of death were cardiovascular, respiratory, and anaphylactic. Unfortunately, specific details about these deaths and their temporal relationship to the plasmapheresis procedure are not provided. In his review, Huestis (1) calculated an estimated three deaths per 10,000 procedures.

In a review of 6200 treatments, Aufeuvre et al (2,3) reported a total of seven deaths. Causes of death included nonhemodynamic pulmonary edema (FFP replacement), cardiac dysrhythmia, hemo-dynamic pulmonary edema, and pulmonary embolism. In an extensive review of several large series, involving over 15,000 treatments, we found a total of eight deaths, for a calculated incidence of 0.05% (4).

REFERENCES

1. Huestis DW. Mortality in therapeutic haemapheresis. Lancet 1983;1:1043. Letter.
2. Aufeuvre JP, Morin-Hertel F, Cohen-Solal M, Lefloch A, Baudelot J. Hazards of plasma exchange. In: Sieberth HG, ed. Plasma exchange. Stuttgart, Germany: FK Schattauer Verlag, 1980:149–157.
3. Aufeuvre JP, Mortin-Hertel F, Cohen-Solal M, Lefloch A, Baudelot J. Clinical tolerance and hazards of plasma exchanges: a study of 6200 plasma exchanges in 1033 patients. In: Beyer JH, Burgerg H, Fuchs C, Nagel GA, eds. Plasmapheresis in immunology and oncology. Basel, Switzerland: Karger, 1982: 65–77.
4. Mokrzycki MH, Kaplan AA. Therapeutic plasma exchange: complications and management. Am J Kidney Dis 1994;23: 817–827.

Drug Removal

5

In sharp contrast with what is known about drug kinetics during hemodialysis (1), there is little published information regarding the removal of therapeutic agents by therapeutic plasma exchange (TPE). During plasma exchange, alterations in plasma drug levels are most dependent on the percentage of protein binding and the volume of distribution (2–4). Thus, a drug with a high percentage of protein binding and a relatively modest volume of distribution (<0.3 L/kg) will have the greatest likelihood of being removed by TPE. Using first-order kinetics and assuming the simplest case, the volume of plasma exchanged during a TPE treatment would have to equal 0.7 times the volume of distribution of a drug to remove 50% of its total body burden or 1.4 times the drug's volume of distribution to remove 75% of its total body burden (see Chap. 2). Thus, a TPE treatment would have to exchange 7 liters of plasma to remove 50% of a drug whose volume of distribution is a modest 0.15 L/kg (~10 liters in a 70-kg patient). Given this basic tenet, even a drug with a percentage protein binding of over 90% would be minimally removed if its volume of distribution was at least 0.6 L/kg (≥42 liters in a 70-kg patient). It is therefore not surprising that a 3- or 4-liter TPE treatment is not a widely used means of blood purification for the treatment of drug intoxications, despite the fact that many drugs are very highly protein bound (see Chap. 9 and Chap. 15).

An example of the type of information required to adequately assess the effect of TPE on a given drug is given in Table 5-1. Of note is that the total amount removed is easily calculated by multiplying the drug concentration in the removed plasma by its total volume. Of equal interest is that the post-treatment levels

Table 5-1. Drug Removal During Plasma Exchange

Drug	Serum Levels		Total Amount Removed	V_e/(EPV)	AVD
	Pre-Rx	Post-RX			
				liters	
Vitamin B$_{12}$, μg/L	396	197	890 μg	3/(3.4)	4.5
Phenytoin, mg/L (total)	11	8	29 mg	3/(2.3)	10
Phenytoin, mg/L (free)	0.9	0.6	1.9 mg	3/(2.3)	6
Phenobarbital, mg/L	17	11	45 mg	3/(2.3)	8

Rx, treatment; V_e, volume exchanged; EPV, estimated plasma volume; AVD, apparent volume of distribution.
SOURCE: Reproduced by permission from Kaplan AA, Halley SE. Plasma exchange with a rotating filter. Kidney Int 1990;38:160–166.

may increase rapidly as re-equilibration occurs between the extra-vascular compartments (interstitial, intracellular, intramembranous, etc) and the plasma.

Although definitive data regarding drug kinetics during TPE are limited and often reported in a variety of ways, results obtained for several drugs are reviewed in the following paragraphs. In any event, because of the large variability in drug kinetics between individuals, **it is recommended that, when possible, all daily drug dosing should be administered after the TPE treatment**. Because so few drugs have been studied in a formal manner, Table 5-2 lists several drugs that have both a high percentage of protein binding and a modest volume of distribution. As noted above, these characteristics would suggest that these drugs are likely to be significantly affected by TPE, either by a single treatment or during a series of closely spaced treatments.

Specific Drugs

Many indications for plasma exchange involve the concomitant administration of steroids and immunosuppressive medication. **Prednisone** has a relatively large volume of distribution (1 L/kg), and despite a protein binding of between 70 and 95%, neither it nor its metabolite, **prednisolone**, is significantly removed by plasma exchange and supplemental dosing after TPE has been found to be unnecessary (5). One can anticipate minimal removal

Table 5-2. Drugs with a High Percentage of Protein Binding and Modest Volume of Distribution

	% Protein Binding	Volume of Distribution V_d (L/kg)
ASA	50–90	0.1–0.2
Cefazolin	80	0.13–0.22
Cefotetan	85	0.15
Ceftriaxone	90	0.12–0.18
Chlorpropamide	72–96	0.09–0.27
Diclofenac	>99	0.12–0.17
Dicloxacillin	95	0.16
Glyburide	99	0.16–0.3
Heparin	>90	0.06–0.1
Ibuprofen	99	0.15–0.17
Indomethacin	99	0.12
Ketorolac	>99	0.13–0.25
Naproxen	99	0.10
Probenecid	85–95	0.15
Sodium valproate	90	0.19–0.23
Streptokinase	?	0.02–0.08
Tolbutamide	95–97	0.10–0.15
Warfarin	97–99	0.11–0.15

In general, drugs with a high percentage of protein binding and a modest volume of distribution are likely to be removed by plasma exchange.
SOURCE: Data from references 1, 3, and 4.

of **cyclophosphamide** with TPE, because the percentage of protein binding is low (12%) and the volume of distribution is relatively large (0.8 L/kg) (3). **Azathioprine** is approximately 30% protein bound, with a volume of distribution of 0.6 L/kg, suggesting minimal removal by TPE.

Most **aminoglycosides** have a low degree of protein binding (<5%) and a volume of distribution approximating 0.25 L/kg; thus, one would not predict a substantial removal by TPE. Predictably, only 7 to 10% of a 100-mg dose of **tobramycin** was removed after two TPE treatments equaling 1700 and 2170 mL (6). Similarly, only 4 to 6% of body stores were removed after single TPE treatments of 1725 and 2057 mL (3).

Phenytoin has a variable volume of distribution of between 0.5 and 1 L/kg and has a substantial intraerythrocytic distribution. Lui and Rubenstein (7) reported that approximately 10% of total body stores were removed during TPE treatments of 5.6 and 6.1 liters, suggesting that a post-treatment supplement may be required. Depending on initial serum concentrations, which varied between 8 and 17 µg/mL, the total amount removed ranged from 42 to 93 mg per treatment. Our own data, obtained after a 3-liter exchange, demonstrated a net 30-mg removal (see Table 5-1) (2).

Digoxin, with an enormous volume of distribution (5 to 8 L/kg) and a modest degree of protein binding (20 to 30%), is predictably unaffected by TPE (3), but removal of digibind-bound drug may be enhanced in patients with renal failure (8). **Digitoxin** has a greater degree of protein binding (94%), but its volume of distribution, although far less than that of digoxin (0.6 L/kg), is still too great to allow for a substantial net removal, and TPE has not been found to significantly lower its total body stores (3). Despite the modest net removal, TPE may still be useful as a treatment for intoxications because cardiac toxicity may be reduced because of the rapid lowering of serum levels (9,10) (see Chap. 15).

Twenty-five percent of the active hormone, **thyroxine**, circulates in the intravascular compartment and is 99% bound to serum protein, leading to the use of TPE to treat thyroid storm when conventional methods have failed (11).

In agreement with its high percentage of protein binding (up to 90%) and its modest volume of distribution (0.1 to 0.2 L/kg), TPE exchanges equaling 20 mL/kg have been found to remove substantial amounts of **acetylsalicylic acid** (3). Although its large volume of distribution (2.8 to 4 L/kg) would suggest that net removal would be minimal, TPE has been reported to reduce the half-life of **propranolol** (90 to 96% protein bound) by approximately 75% (12). **Vancomycin** is only 10 to 50% protein bound and has a volume of distribution that ranges between 0.5 and 1.1 L/kg. A one plasma volume exchange has been found to remove only 6% of total body stores, with a substantial post-treatment rebound suggesting a substantial redistribution (13).

REFERENCES

1. Bennet WM, Aronoff GR, Golper TA, Morrison G, Singer I, Brater DC. Drug prescribing in renal failure. 2nd ed. Philadelphia: American College of Physicians, 1991.
2. Kaplan AA, Halley SE. Plasma exchange with a rotating filter. Kidney Int 1990;38:160–166.

3. Sketris IS, Parker WA, Jones JV. Effect of plasma exchange on drug removal. In: Valbonesi M, Pineda AA, Biggs JC, eds. Therapeutic hemapheresis. Milano, Italy: Wichtig Editore, 1986:15–20.

4. Jones JV. The effect of plasmapheresis on therapeutic drugs. Dial Transplant 1985;14:225–226.

5. Stigelman WH, Henry DH, Talbert RL, Townsend RJ. Removal of prednisone and prednisolone by plasma exchange. Clin Pharmacol 1984;3:402–407.

6. Appelgate R, Schwartz D, Bennett WM. Removal of tobramycin during plasma exchange therapy. Ann Intern Med 1981;94:820–821.

7. Liu E, Rubenstein M. Phenytoin removal by plasmapheresis in thrombotic thrombocytopenic purpura. Clin Pharmacol Ther 1982;31:762–765.

8. Rabetoy GM, Price CA, Findlay JW, Sailstad JM. Treatment of digoxin intoxication in a renal failure patient with digoxin-specific antibody fragments and plasmapheresis. Am J Nephrol 1990;10:518–521.

9. Peters U, Risler T, Grabenese B. Digitoxin elimination by plasma separation. In: Sieberth HG, ed. Plasma exchange: plasmapheresis-plasmaseparation. Stuttgart: FK Schattauer Verlag, 1980:365–368.

10. Arsac Ph, Barret L, Chenais F, Debru JL, Faure J. Digitoxin intoxication treated by plasma exchange. In: Sieberth HG, ed. Plasma exchange: plasmapheresis-plasmaseparation. Stuttgart: FK Schattauer Verlag, 1980:369–371.

11. Ashkar FS, Katims RB, Smoak WM, Gilson AJ. Thyroid storm treatment with blood exchange and plasmapheresis. JAMA 1979;214:1275–1279.

12. Talbert RL, Wong YY, Duncan DB. Propranolol plasma concentrations and plasmapheresis. Drug Intell Clin Phram 1981;15:993–996.

13. McClellan SD, Whitaker CH, Friedberg RC. Removal of vancomycin during plasmapheresis. Ann Pharmacother 1997;31:1132–1136.

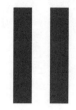

Indications

Introduction to Indications

6

In 1985, the American Medical Association (AMA) council on scientific affairs convened a panel of 10 experts to review the available data on the efficacy of plasma exchange (1). Their assessment assigned each potential indication into one of four categories: (I) standard therapy, acceptable but not mandatory; (II) available evidence tends to favor efficacy: conventional therapy usually tried first; (III) inadequately tested at this time; and (IV) no demonstrated value in controlled trials. Since this AMA review, there have been several well-designed, randomized, controlled trials that have added significant new insight into the proper application of therapeutic plasma exchange. In consideration of these new studies, two subsequent reviews attempted to update the original AMA recommendations (2,3). Added to these updated reviews is a most recent assessment by the American Academy of Neurology (4). A list of the original AMA indications, updated and modified by the three subsequent reviews, appears in Table 6-1.

Table 6-1. Indications for TPE

	Reference and year			
	1 1986	2 1993	3 1994	4 1996
Neurologic diseases				
Guillain-Barré syndrome	I	I	I	Est
Myasthenia gravis	I	I	I	Est
Chronic inflammatory demyelinating polyneuropathy	III	I	I	Est
Paraprotein-associated polyneuropathy	nl	II	nl	Est
Multiple sclerosis	II	III	III	Pos
Eaton-Lambert syndrome	nl	I	nl	Pos
Stiff-man syndrome	nl	nl	nl	Invest
Amyotrophic lateral sclerosis	IV	IV	IV	nl
Neuromyotonia	nl	nl	nl	Invest
Acute disseminated encephalomyelitis	nl	nl	nl	Invest
Refsum's disease	nl	I	nl	Invest
Sensorineural hearing loss	nl	nl	nl	nl
Hematologic disorders				
Hyperviscosity syndrome	I	I	I	
Cryoglobulinemia	II	I	I	
Thrombotic thrombocytopenic purpura/hemolytic uremic syndrome	I nl	I II	I II	
Idiopathic thrombocytopenic purpura	III	III	III	
Post-transfusion purpura	II	I	I	
Autoimmune hemolytic anemia	III	III	III	
Maternal-fetal incompatibility-Rh disease	II	III	nl	
Removal of factor VIII inhibitors	II	II	III	
Metabolic disorders				
Hypercholesterolemia	II	I–II	I	
Hypertriglyceridemia	nl	nl	nl	
Pruritis associated with cholestasis	II	nl	nl	
Hepatic failure	III	III	nl	
Graves' disease and thyroid storm	I	III	III	
Insulin receptor antibodies	nl	nl	nl	
Dermatologic disorders				
Pemphigus vulgaris	III	II	nl	
Bullous pemphigus	nl	II	nl	
Toxic epidermal necrolysis (Lyell's syndrome)	nl	nl	nl	
Porphyria cutanea tarda	nl	nl	nl	
Psoriasis	III	IV	IV	

Table 6-1. *Continued*

	Reference and year			
	1 **1986**	**2** **1993**	**3** **1994**	**4** **1996**
Rheumatologic disorders				
Systemic lupus erythematosus	II	II	nl	
Antiphospholipid syndrome (lupus anticoagulant)	nl	nl	nl	
Scleroderma	III	III	III	
Rheumatoid arthritis and rheumatoid vasculitis	II	III	IV and II	
Vasculitis	II	II	II	
Polymyositis/dermatomyositis	III	III/IV	IV	
Renal disease				
Goodpasture's syndrome	I	I	I	
Rapidly progressive glomerulonephritis	I	II	II	
Multiple myeloma, "cast nephropathy"	II	II	nl	
Henoch-Schonlein purpura/IgA nephropathy	II	nl	nl	
Focal segmental glomerulosclerosis: recurrence post-transplant	nl	nl	nl	
Renal allograft rejection	II	IV	IV	
Removal of cytotoxic antibodies in the transplant candidate	nl	nl	nl	
Indications for TPE in the ICU				
Fulminant systemic meningococcemia	nl	nl	nl	
Endotoxemia	nl	nl	nl	
Burn shock	III	nl	nl	
Human immunodeficiency virus	III	nl	nl	
Immune thrombocytopenic purpura	nl	II	nl	
Thrombotic thrombocytopenic purpura	nl	I	nl	
Peripheral neuropathy	nl	I	nl	
Intoxications	I	II	II	
Arsine				
Carbamazepine				
Cisplatin				
Digitoxin				
Digoxin				
Diltiazem				
Mushroom poisoning		II		
Paraquat		II		
Parathion		II		

Table 6-1. *Continued*

	Reference and year			
	1 1986	2 1993	3 1994	4 1996
Phenylbutazone				
Phenytoin				
Quinine				
Sodium chlorate		II		
Theophylline				
Thyroxine				
Tricyclic antidepressant				
Vincristine				

Rating: I, standard therapy, acceptable but not mandatory; II, available evidence tends to favor efficacy: conventional therapy usually tried first; III, inadequately tested at this time; IV, no demonstrated value in controlled trials. Est, established therapy; Invest, investigational; Pos, possibly useful; nl, not listed; ICU; intensive care unit.

REFERENCES

1. American Medical Association Council on Scientific Affairs. Current status of therapeutic plasmapheresis. JAMA 1985;253: 819–825.
2. Strauss RG, Ciavarella D, Gilcher RO, et al. An overview of current management. J Clin Apheresis 1993;8:189–194.
3. Leitman SF, Ciavarella D, McLeod B, Owen H, Price T, Sniecinski I. Guidelines for therapeutic hemapheresis. Bethesda, MD: American Association of Blood Banks, Revised 1994.
4. Assessment of plasmapheresis. Report of the Therapeutics and Technology Assessment Subcommittee of the American Academy of Neurology. Neurology 1996;47:840–843.

Neurologic Disorders

7

Guillain-Barré Syndrome   91
Myasthenia Gravis   94
Chronic Inflammatory Demyelinating Polyneuropathy   96
Paraprotein-Associated Polyneuropathy   98
  Monoclonal Gammopathy of Undetermined Significance   98
  Waldenström's Macroglobulinemia   98
  Cryoglobulinemia   99
Multiple Sclerosis   100
Eaton-Lambert Syndrome   102
Stiff-Man Syndrome   103
Amyotrophic Lateral Sclerosis   104
Neuromyotonia (Isaacs' Syndrome)   105
Acute Disseminated Encephalomyelitis   105
Sensorineural Hearing Loss: Immune-Mediated Inner Ear Disease   106
Refsum's Disease   107

In the United States, neurologic diseases represent the most common indication for therapeutic plasma exchange (TPE) (1). In 1996, the American Academy of Neurology reviewed the available evidence and concluded that TPE has a definite role in the management of Guillain-Barré syndrome, chronic inflammatory demyelinating polyneuropathies (CIDP), polyneuropathies associated with monoclonal gammopathies of unknown significance, myasthenia gravis, and Eaton-Lambert syndrome (Table 7-1) (2). TPE was also considered as having a possible role in the treatment of Refsum's disease, acquired neuromyotonia, stiff-man syndrome, cryoglobulinemic polyneuropathy, central nervous system (CNS) lupus, acute disseminated encephalomyelitis (ADEM), and multiple sclerosis. In contrast, the Academy concluded that TPE had no role in the treatment of amyotrophic lateral sclerosis (ALS) or parane-

Table 7-1.   Neurologic Indications for TPE

	Reference and year			
	1 1986	2 1993	3 1994	4 1996
Neurologic diseases				
Guillain-Barré syndrome	I	I	I	Est
Myasthenia gravis	I	I	I	Est
CIDP	III	I	I	Est
Paraprotein-associated polyneuropathy	nl	II	nl	Est
Multiple sclerosis	II	III	III	Pos
Eaton-Lambert syndrome	nl	I	nl	Pos
Stiff-man syndrome	nl	nl	nl	Invest
Amyotrophic lateral sclerosis	IV	IV	IV	nl
Neuromyotonia	nl	nl	nl	Invest
Acute disseminated encephalomyelitis	nl	nl	nl	Invest
Sensorineural hearing loss	nl	nl	nl	nl
Refsum's disease	nl	I	nl	Invest

I, standard therapy, acceptable but not mandatory; II, available evidence tends to favor efficacy: conventional therapy usually tried first; III, inadequately tested at this time; IV, no demonstrated value in controlled trials; Est, established therapy; Invest, investigational; Pos, possibly useful; nl, not listed.

REFERENCES: 1. American Medical Association Council on Scientific Affairs. Current status of therapeutic plasmapheresis. JAMA 1985;253:819–825.
2. Strauss RG, Ciavarella D, Gilcher RO, et al. An overview of current management. J Clin Apheresis 1993;8:189–194.
3. Leitman SF, Ciavarella D, McLeod B, et al. Guidelines for therapeutic hemapheresis. Bethesda, MD: American Association of Blood Banks, Revised 1994.
4. Assessment of plasmapheresis. Report of the Therapeutics and Technology Assessment Subcommittee of the American Academy of Neurology. Neurology 1996;47:840–843.

oplastic syndromes with circulating autoantibodies. The separate sections provided in this chapter review the available data and provide concise recommendations on how to prescribe TPE for each given disease entity.

Aside from the above-mentioned assessment by the American Academy of Neurology, there have been several indepth reviews of the use of TPE in neurologic diseases (3–6).

REFERENCES

1. Malchesky PS, Bambauer R, Horiuchi T, Kaplan AA, Sakurada Y, Samuelsson G. Apheresis technologies: an international perspective. Artif Organs 1995;19:315–323.

2. Assessment of plasmapheresis. Report of the Therapeutics and Technology Assessment Subcommittee of the American Academy of Neurology. Neurology 1996;47:840–843.

3. NIH Consensus Conference. The utility of therapeutic plasmapheresis for neurological disorders. JAMA 1986;256:1333–1337.

4. Lisak RP. Plasma exchange in neurologic diseases. Arch Neurol 1984;41:654–657.

5. Ciavarella D, Wuest D, Strauss RG, Gilcher RO, Kasprisin DO, Kiprov DD, Klein HG, McLeod BC. Management of neurologic disorders. J Clin Apheresis 1993;8:242–257.

6. Thornton CA, Griggs RC. Plasma exchange and intravenous immunoglobulin treatment of neuromuscular disease. Ann Neurol 1994;35:260–268.

GUILLAIN-BARRÉ SYNDROME

Guillain-Barré syndrome is an acute demyelinating neuropathy characterized by bilateral upper and lower extremity muscle weakness, loss of reflexes, and variable degrees of sensory loss. Autonomic dysfunction is common and manifests as arrhythmias, hypertension, and orthostatic hypotension. Bulbar involvement with respiratory failure is a major cause of morbidity and mortality, and elective intubation is recommended when vital capacity is 15 mL/kg or less (1). Two-thirds of cases follow an infection and up to 26% of cases may have evidence of a recent infection with *Campylobacter jejuni* enteritis (2,3). Other associated infections include human immunodeficiency virus (HIV), cytomegalovirus, and Epstein-Barr virus. In other cases, there may be an underlying disease such as systemic lupus erythematosus, Hodgkin's disease, or sarcoidosis. Inoculation for swine influenza has also been implicated (1). Diagnosis is supported by the existence of an "albuminocytologic dissociation" in the cerebrospinal fluid, with findings of increased protein with few cells. Rationale for TPE therapy is supported by reports of antibodies directed against various constituents of peripheral myelin (1). The most compelling evidence for the efficacy of TPE comes from a multicenter trial involving 21 medical centers coordinated by Johns Hopkins University (Table 7-2) (4). This study randomized 245 patients to be treated with either supportive therapy or plasma exchange. Those receiving TPE had a substantially shortened duration of motor weakness (29 versus 40 days) and, for those developing respiratory failure after randomization, a shorter period of ventilatory support (24 versus 48 days). Based on the results of

Table 7-2. The Guillain-Barré Syndrome Study Group: Controlled Trial of TPE

	TPE	Control
Number of patients	122[a]	123
Number of patients on respirator	57	52
Time to improve 1 grade (days)	19	40[b]
Mean change in grade after 4 weeks	1.1	0.4[b]
Time on respirator (days)	24	48[b]

Neurologic grading scale: 0, healthy; 1, minor signs or symptoms; 2, able to walk 5 meters unaided; 3, able to walk 5 meters assisted; 4, bed- or chairbound; 5, requires assisted ventilation; 6, deceased.
[a] twelve patients did not complete TPE regimen.
[b] $p < 0.01$ when compared with TPE-treated group.
SOURCE: Adapted from the report of The Guillain-Barré Syndrome Study Group. Plasmapheresis and acute Guillain-Barré syndrome. Neurology 1985;35:1096–1104.

this study and two other randomized controlled trials (5,6), a recent assessment by the American Academy of Neurology gave plasmapheresis a strong positive recommendation as an established therapy (7). TPE is recommended for patients with severe weakness, which may include inability to walk and difficulty breathing or other signs of bulbar insufficiency, including loss of gag reflex or difficulty swallowing (8,9). **Successful treatment has been obtained with a total of three to five one–plasma volume exchanges delivered over a 7- to 14-day period (2) or a total of 200 to 250 mL/kg of plasma exchanged over four to six treatments (1).**

Relapse after early improvement has been described, suggesting that TPE may have been discontinued prematurely. If this type of biphasic illness is noted, retreatment with TPE should be considered (9). **Successful retreatment has been achieved with three to five TPE treatments over 5 to 10 days with a total exchange volume ranging from 11.5 to 14 liters (10).**

A recent Dutch study compared the accepted TPE regimen with the infusion of intravenous immunoglobulins (IVIG), demonstrating a better or at least equal outcome with IVIG (11). An accompanying review found these results difficult to interpret because the patients treated with TPE did less well than expected (1). Most recently, a comprehensive comparison of IVIG and TPE for neurologic diseases suggested that those receiving IVIG may have a tendency to relapse (12). Our own experience is anecdotal, but we have had patients respond to TPE after failing to respond to IVIG.

REFERENCES

1. Ropper AH. The Guillain-Barré syndrome. N Engl J Med 1992;326:1130–1135.
2. Rees JH, Soudain SE, Gregson NA, Hughes RAC. *Campylobacter jejuni* infection and Guillain-Barré syndrome. N Engl J Med 1995;333:1374–1379.
3. Bolton CF. The changing concepts of Guillain-Barré syndrome. N Engl J Med 1995;333:1415–1416. Editorial.
4. The Guillain-Barré Syndrome Study Group. Plasmapheresis and acute Guillain-Barré syndrome. Neurology 1985;35:1096–1104.
5. Osterman PO, Fagius J, Lundemo G, Pihlstedt P, Pirskanen R, Siden A, Safwenberg J. Beneficial effects of plasma exchange in acute inflammatory polyradiculoneuropathy. Lancet 1984;2:1296–1299.
6. French Cooperative Group on Plasma Exchange in Guillain-Barré syndrome. Efficiency of plasma exchange in Guillain-Barré syndrome: role of replacement fluids. Ann Neurol 1987;22:753–761.
7. Assessment of plasmapheresis. Report of the Therapeutics and Technology Assessment Subcommittee of the American Academy of Neurology. Neurology 1996;47:840–843.
8. NIH Consensus Conference. The utility of therapeutic plasmapheresis for neurological disorders. JAMA 1986;256:1333–1337.
9. Ciavarella D, Wuest D, Strauss RG, Gilcher RO, Kasprisin DO, Kiprov DD, Klein HG, McLeod BC. Management of neurologic disorders. J Clin Apheresis 1993;8:242–257.
10. Ropper AH, Albers JW, Addison R. Limited relapse in Guillain-Barré syndrome after plasma exchange. Arch Neurol 1988;45:314–315.
11. van der Meche FGA, Schmitz PIM, the Dutch Guillain-Barré Study Group. A randomized trial comparing intravenous immune globulin and plasma exchange in Guillain-Barré syndrome. N Engl J Med 1992;326:1123–1129.
12. Thorton CA, Griggs RC. Plasma exchange and intravenous immunoglobulin treatment of neuromuscular disease. Ann Neurol 1994;35:260–268.

MYASTHENIA GRAVIS

Myasthenia gravis is an antibody-mediated autoimmune disease in which the neuromuscular weakness can be attributed to the presence of anti-acetylcholine receptor (AChR) antibodies. Weakness of the proximal muscle groups and those of the eyes, mouth, and throat is predominant. The disease is often associated with thymic abnormalities, such as hyperplasia or thymoma. There may also be other autoimmune phenomena. Diagnostic tests include an increase in muscle strength after the use of cholinergic drugs (edrophonium) and diminishing amplitude of evoked muscle action potentials after repeated electrical stimulation.

Standard therapy involves anticholinergic drugs and often includes some form of immunosuppressive therapy such as steroids, cyclophosphamide, or azathioprine. Although several uncontrolled trials suggest that TPE can induce short-term improvement and numerous anecdotal reports describe dramatic post-treatment results (1–5), there has never been a controlled trial of TPE for myasthenia gravis. Nonetheless, an NIH consensus panel (6) concluded that TPE can be useful in increasing muscle strength in the pre- and post-thymectomy period and in decreasing symptoms during the initiation of immunosuppressive therapy and during an acute crisis. More recently, the American Academy of Neurology concluded that plasmapheresis was an established therapy for myasthenia gravis that could be given a "positive" recommendation (7). Although seemingly contradictory, TPE has also been found to be beneficial in four of eight patients with seronegative myasthenia gravis, a condition that can occur in up to 18.5% of cases (8). Possible explanations for seronegativity include the inability of the assay to detect the antibody, relative antigen excess, and the existence of antibodies that may be directed against a different antigenic determinant of the neuromuscular junction.

For acute symptoms unresponsive to conventional therapy, a reasonable treatment prescription is four to eight TPE treatments over a 1- to 2-week period. In seriously ill patients, treatments should be given daily or every other day (9). Each treatment should equal one plasma volume, which can be replaced with albumin. If the patient is in the immediate pre- or post-thymectomy period, a partial replacement of approximately 1 liter of fresh frozen plasma (FFP), given toward the end of each treatment, should help minimize the expected depletion coagulopathy. A small number of patients whose symp-

Table 7-3. Observed and Predicted Decline in Anti-Acetylcholine Receptor Antibody

Date	Pre-RX	Post-RX	V_e	EPV	V_e/EPV	% Decline Actual	% Decline Predicted
	nmol/L		*L*				
3/23	5.6	1.5	4	2.8	1.43	73	76
3/24	2.4	<0.5[a]	4	2.9	1.38	79	75
3/25	<0.5	<0.5	4	2.9	1.38	NA	75
4/12	6.9	3.7	1.2[b]	2.8	0.41	46[b]	35
4/13	5.9	1.0	5	2.8	1.79	83	83

Predicted values were obtained using first-order kinetics and assumed the apparent volume of distribution of the antibody to be equal to the EPV.
[a] This value was considered to be 0.5 for the purpose of calculation.
[b] This procedure was terminated prematurely due to access difficulties. Large amounts of saline flushes may have contributed to the measured decline in post-treatment levels.
V_e, volume exchanged; EPV, estimated plasma volume.
NA, not applicable, due to the unmeasurable levels.
SOURCE: Reproduced by permission from Kaplan AA, Halley SE. Plasma exchange with a rotating filter. Kidney Int 1990;38:160–166.

toms are improved by TPE will experience clinical deterioration when weaned from the treatments. Under these conditions, chronic intermittent TPE, in conjunction with azathioprine, has been successfully used for over 4 years. **Initial intertreatment intervals were 3 to 6 weeks, ultimately averaging from 6.8 to 9.2 exchanges per year.** Determination of the required intertreatment interval should be by the reappearance of symptoms and not by the level of AChR antibody (10).

Although levels of AChR antibody are unlikely to be immediately available to monitor therapy, retrospective comparison between observed and expected declines in AChR antibodies reveals an excellent correlation with the calculated kinetics of total IgG removal (Table 7-3) (11).

REFERENCES

1. Dau PC, Lindstrom JM, Cassel CK, Denys EH, Shev EE, Spitler LE. Plasmapheresis and immunosuppressive drug therapy in myasthenia gravis. N Engl J Med 1997;297:1134–1140.

2. Newsom-Davis J, Wilson SG, Vincent A, Ward CD. Long-term effects of repeated plasma exchange in myasthenia gravis. Lancet 1979;1:464–468.

3. Behan PO, Shakir RA, Simpson JA, Burnett AK, Allan TL, Haase G. Plasma-exchange combined with immunosuppressive therapy in myasthenia gravis. Lancet 1979;2:438–440.

4. Seybold ME. Plasmapheresis in myasthenia gravis. Ann NY Acad Sci 1987;505:584–587.

5. Levin KH, Richman DP. Myasthenia gravis. Clin Aspects Autoimmun 1989;4:23–31.

6. NIH Consensus Conference. The utility of therapeutic plasmapheresis for neurological disorders. JAMA 1986;256:1333–1337.

7. Assessment of plasmapheresis. Report of the Therapeutics and Technology Assessment Subcommittee of the American Academy of Neurology. Neurology 1996;47:840–843.

8. Soliven BC, Lange DJ, Penn AS, et al. Seronegative myasthenia gravis. Neurol 1988;38:514–517.

9. Ciavarella D, Wuest D, Strauss RG, Gilcher RO, Kasprisin DO, Kiprov DD, Klein HG, McLeod BC. Management of neurologic disorders. J Clin Apheresis 1993;8:242–257.

10. Rodnitzky RL, Bosch EP. Chronic long-interval plasma exchange in myasthenia gravis. Arch Neurol 1984;41:715–717.

11. Kaplan AA, Halley SE. Plasma exchange with a rotating filter. Kidney Int 1990;38:160–166.

CHRONIC INFLAMMATORY DEMYELINATING POLYNEUROPATHY

CIDP is believed to be an autoimmune disease characterized by a progressive or relapsing course, symmetric motor or motor and sensory loss, hypo- or areflexia, and the absence of systemic symptoms. A disease duration greater than 2 months distinguishes it from Guillain-Barré syndrome. Abnormalities supporting the diagnoses include elevated cerebrospinal fluid protein, severe slowing of nerve conduction velocity, and segmental demyelinization on nerve biopsy. The condition can progress to severe disability or death (1).

Conventional therapy may include corticosteroids and other immunosuppressive agents, including azathioprine, cyclophosphamide, and cyclosporin A. Although several uncontrolled studies have reported potential benefit for plasma exchange therapy (2–5), the most convincing data come from a randomized, sham-controlled trial of severely affected patients (6). **Treatment prescription was for two plasma exchange procedures per week for 3 weeks. Each exchange averaged 47 mL/kg body weight or a mean 3.5 liters.** Replacement was with albumin. Approximately one-third of those treated with TPE responded with improvement in neurologic disability scores and in nerve conduction. There was no way to identify the responders. In those patients who responded, improvement generally began to fade within 10 to 14 days after treatment was discontinued, suggesting that a maintenance treatment schedule may be required to sustain remission. Indeed, Feasby et al (3), in a preliminary report, concluded that **maintenance of neurologic improvement required TPE to be performed in a schedule ranging from weekly to every 3 weeks for up to 60 months.**

A recent assessment by the American Academy of Neurology gave TPE a "strong positive recommendation" as an established therapy for CIDP (7).

REFERENCES

1. Mendell JR. Chronic inflammatory demyelinating polyradiculoneuropathy. Annu Rev Med 1993;44:211–219.
2. Server AC, Lefkowith J, Braine H, McKhann GM. Treatment of chronic relapsing inflammatory polyradiculoneuropathy by plasma exchange. Ann Neurol 1979;6:258–261.
3. Feasby TE, Hahn AF, Brown WF. Long term plasmapheresis in chronic progressive demyelinating polyneuropathy. Ann Neurol 1983;14:122. Abstract.
4. Toyka KV, Augspach R, Paulus W, Grabensee B, Hein D. Plasma exchange in polyradiculoneuropathy. Ann Neurol 1980;8:205–206. Letter.
5. Fowler H, Vulp M, Marks G, et al. Recovery from chronic progressive polyneuropathy after treatment with plasma exchange. Lancet 1979;2:1193.
6. Dyck PJ, Daube J, O'Brien P, Pineda A, Low PA, Windebank AJ, Swanson C. Plasma exchange in chronic inflammatory demyelinating polyradiculoneuropathy. N Engl J Med 1986; 314:461–465.
7. Assessment of plasmapheresis. Report of the Therapeutics and Technology Assessment Subcommittee of the American Academy of Neurology. Neurology 1996;47:840–843.

PARAPROTEIN-ASSOCIATED POLYNEUROPATHY

Monoclonal Gammopathy of Undetermined Significance

The presence of monoclonal antibodies may be associated with a demyelinating process characterized by a mixed sensorimotor neuropathy with distal weakness, tremor, ataxia, and loss of proprioception. In most patients, the antibody is IgM, but IgA- and IgG-associated neuropathies have also been described. The neuropathy seems to be associated with the binding of the antibody to certain constituents of peripheral myelin such as myelin-associated glycoprotein or glycolipids. In one clinicopathologic study, IgM and activated complement components were demonstrated in localized areas of demyelination, strongly suggesting a pathogenetic role for these immunoglobulins (1). The removal of these antibodies is the rationale for TPE treatments. In a randomized, sham-controlled trial of patients with MGUS-related neuropathies, patients receiving TPE had significantly improved neurologic disability scores and muscle action potentials when compared with the sham-treated patients (2). Sham-treated patients who were subsequently treated with TPE showed similar improvement. Those patients with IgA- or IgG-related neuropathies received the greatest benefit. **Treatment prescription was two plasma exchange treatments per week for 3 weeks. Each exchange averaged 47 mL/kg or approximately 3.5 liters. Replacement was with albumin.** In a recent technology assessment, the American Academy of Neurology concluded that for patients with IgA- or IgG-related neuropathies, TPE could be considered as "established" therapy (3). For patients with IgM-related neuropathies, TPE could be considered as "possibly useful."

Waldenström's Macroglobulinemia

Peripheral neuropathy occurs in about 5% of cases of Waldenström's macroglobulinemia. Some cases may involve direct toxicity of the macroglobulin to the myelin sheath, in which case the peripheral neuropathy may antedate the hematologic symptoms by several years and the serum levels of monoclonal IgM may be low. In other cases, the IgM may not react directly with myelin sheath components and neuropathy may be associated with perivascular lymphoplasmacytic infiltrates (4). The hyperviscosity syndrome (see Chap. 8) associated with macroglobulinemia may also cause peripheral neuropathy by inducing microvascular ischemia. Two series of TPE treatments were reported by the same authors (4). In one series, improvement in neuropathy and long-lasting decreases in IgM levels were obtained in three of six patients with alkalating agents and intermittent TPE. In the other series, a more extensive TPE prescription produced improvement in four of five patients (4). **In neither series was the TPE prescription described, but it would be reasonable to prescribe therapy in a manner shown to be effective in MGUS-related neuropathy (see above).**

Cryoglobulinemia

Peripheral neuropathy occurs in 7 to 15% of patients with cryoglobulinemia, presenting most often with a symmetric, subacute, distal, sensorimotor polyneuropathy. Pathogenesis may involve immunologic-mediated demyelination, microcirculatory occlusion, or vasculitis of the vasa nervosum (5,6). The neuropathy may be vasculitic in nature and respond completely to TPE (6). **Successful treatment has been achieved with three TPE procedures performed in rapid succession, followed by a maintenance schedule of one treatment every 8 to 10 weeks (7).**

In a recent assessment, the American Academy of Neurology concluded that TPE may have a role in the treatment of cryoglobulinemic polyneuropathy but that the evidence was insufficient to determine the appropriateness of the indication (3).

REFERENCES

1. Monaco S, Bonetti B, Ferrari S, et al. Complement-mediated demyelinisation in patients with IgM monoclonal gammopathy and polyneuropathy. N Engl J Med 1990;322:649–652.
2. Dyck PJ, Low PA, Windebank AJ, et al. Plasma exchange in polyneuropathy associated with monoclonal gammopathy of undetermined significance. N Engl J Med 1991;325:1482–1486.
3. Assessment of plasmapheresis. Report of the Therapeutics and Technology Assessment Subcommittee of the American Academy of Neurology. Neurology 1996;47:840–843.
4. Dellagi K, Dupouey P, Brouet JC, Billecocq A, Gomez D, Clauvel JP, Seligmann M. Waldenström's macroglobulinemia and peripheral neuropathy: a clinical and immunologic study. Blood 1983;62:280–285.
5. Malchesky PS, Clough JD. Cryoglobulins: properties, prevalence in disease and removal. Cleve Clin Q 1985;52:175–192.

6. Chad D, Oaruser JM, Bradley WG, Adelman LS, Pinn VM. The pathogenesis of cryoglobulinemic neuropathy. Neurology 1982;32:725–729.

7. Berkman EM, Orlin JB. Use of plasmapheresis and partial plasma exchange in the management of patients with cryoglobulinemia. Transfusion 1980;20:171–178.

MULTIPLE SCLEROSIS

Multiple sclerosis is characterized by scattered areas of demyelination in the CNS. Neurologic deficits consistent with two or more CNS white matter lesions occurring at least 1 month apart are required for the diagnosis. Initial symptoms include asymmetric extremity weakness, vision loss, and paresthesias. The clinical course is often one of relapses and remissions, which in some patients leads to progressive neurologic deterioration. Pathogenesis is unclear but may involve a combination of genetic, environmental, infectious, and autoimmune mechanisms. Classically, the cerebrospinal fluid reveals an elevation of gammaglobulins in an oligoclonal pattern. Lymphocytic invasion into the multiple sclerosis associated plaques, in the absence of an obvious infectious agent, has suggested its autoimmune nature, and TPE has been suggested as a possible treatment.

In 1985, **Khatri et al (1) reported a double-blind, sham-controlled study of 54 patients in which weekly TPE was found to provide improvement in disability scores when added to a regimen of prednisone and low-dose oral cyclophosphamide**. A follow-up evaluation of up to 6 years found the same conclusion and no evidence of major life-threatening complications attributable to the treatment regimen (2). Of note, however, was that the original study was met with considerable skepticism, as reflected in the accompanying editorial, which questioned its use of statistical analysis and pointed out the unpredictable nature of multiple sclerosis and the lack of any objective marker of disease activity (3). Subsequently, a Canadian multi-center cooperative study randomized 168 patients to receive cyclophosphamide and prednisone, with or without weekly TPE or placebo medications and sham TPE (4). After approximately 20 weeks of active treatment, the patients were monitored for disability scores for a mean 30 months of follow-up. Although there was a trend in decreased disability in the TPE group noted at 12, 18, and 24 months of follow-up, the difference was not sustained at 36 months. Although this trial maintained the highest standards of rigor, several reviewers noted that increased supplemental steroids given to the placebo group may have diminished differences between the treatments (5,6). This may seem to be a valid criticism, but the original authors argue that a logical extension of this argument would be that a placebo group given supplemental steroids was able to attain the same results as those treated with an aggressive protocol of TPE, steroids, and cyclophosphamide (7). Perhaps a better criticism is that despite a trend toward improvement lasting up to 24 months, there were no further TPE treatments given after the first 20 weeks. Indeed, the authors of this study clearly state that "it remains possible that a more aggressive or longer course of cyclophosphamide, prednisone and plasma exchange could produce a clinically and statistically significant benefit" (4).

In contrast to the above studies designed to investigate TPE treatment as a strategy for long-term management, a report by Rodriguez et al (8) suggested that TPE may be useful in the treatment of fulminant multiple sclerosis, even without the use of concomitant immunosuppression. Their retrospective analysis describes eight patients unresponsive to high-dose steroid therapy who subsequently demonstrated remarkable improvement after the initiation of TPE. **Successful TPE prescription for these severe episodes was six to nine treatments delivered over 12 to 18 days. The exchange volume was 40 to 50 mL/kg and the replacement fluid was 5% albumin.** In some cases, the neurologic improvement was evident after the second treatment. Most recently, Takahashi et al (9) reported on the successful use of TPE as a "steroid sparing" strategy in the management of childhood multiple sclerosis.

Despite the negative results in the Canadian cooperative study (4) and a similar lack of long-term efficacy reported in another randomized, controlled trial (10), the American Academy of Neurology noted the positive results by Khatri et al (1) and those of Rodriguez et al (8) and concluded that TPE should be considered a "promising" treatment and that it may have a role in selected cases of fulminant multiple sclerosis (11). There is an ongoing double-blind NIH-funded trial of TPE for fulminant multiple sclerosis.

REFERENCES

1. Khatri BO, McQuillen MP, Harrington GJ, Schmoll D, Hoffman RG. Chronic progressive multiple sclerosis: double-

blind controlled study of plasmapheresis in patients taking immunosuppressive drugs. Neurology 1985;35:312–319.

2. Khatri BO, McQuillen MP, Hoffman RG, Harrington GJ, Schmoll D. Plasma exchange in chronic progressive multiple sclerosis: a long term study. Neurology 1991;41:409–414.

3. Weiner HL. An assessment of plasma exchange in progressive multiple sclerosis. Neurology 1985;35:320–322.

4. The Canadian Cooperative Multiple Sclerosis Study Group. The Canadian cooperative trial of cyclophosphamide and plasma exchange in progressive multiple sclerosis. Lancet 1991; 337:441–446.

5. Absher JR. Cyclophosphamide and plasma exchange in multiple sclerosis. Am College of Physicians (ACP) Journal Club 1991;117(suppl 1):11.

6. Ciavarella D, Wuest D, Strauss RG, Gilcher RO, Kasprisin DO, Kiprov DD, Klein HG, McLeod BC. Management of neurologic disorders. J Clin Apheresis 1993;8:242–257.

7. Noseworthy JH, Vandervoort MK, Penman M, Ebers G, Shumak K, Seland TP, Roberts R, Yetisir E, Gent M, Taylor DW. Cyclophosphamide and plasma exchange in multiple sclerosis. Lancet 1991;337:1540–1541. Letter.

8. Rodriguez M, Karnes WE, Bartleson JD, Pineda AA. Plasmapheresis in acute episodes of fulminant CNS inflammatory demyelination. Neurology 1993;43:1100–1104.

9. Takahashi I, Sawaishi Y, Takeda O, Enoki M, Takada G. Childhood multiple sclerosis treated with plasmapheresis. Pediatr Neurol 1997;17:83–87.

10. Weiner HL, Dau PC, Khatri BO, Petajan JH, Birnbaum G, McQuillen MP, Fosburg MT, Feldstein M, Orav EJ. Double-blind study of true vs. sham plasma exchange in patients treated with immunosuppression of acute attacks of multiple sclerosis. Neurology 1989;39:1143–1149.

11. Assessment of plasmapheresis. Report of the Therapeutics and Technology Assessment Subcommittee of the American Academy of Neurology. Neurology 1996;47:840–843.

EATON-LAMBERT SYNDROME

Eaton-Lambert syndrome is a myasthenic-like disorder that can be idiopathic or cancer related. The syndrome is believed to be the result of an antibody-mediated blockage of acetylcholine release by the presynaptic nerve terminal, and calcium channel antibodies have recently been identified (1). Dau and Denys (2) described clinical and electromyographic improvement with either TPE alone or in combination with prednisone and azathioprine. Despite a lack of any controlled trial, TPE with azathioprine and prednisone has been accepted as standard therapy (3,4). **The recommended TPE prescription is a once weekly schedule of 8 to 10 treatments exchanging 45 to 55 mL/kg.**

Citing positive evidence in case-controlled studies and consensus in expert opinion, a recent assessment of the American Academy of Neurology concluded that TPE was a "promising" treatment for Eaton-Lambert syndrome (5).

REFERENCES

1. Lennon VA, Kryzer TJ, Griesmann GE, O'Suilleabhain PE, Windebank AJ, Woppmann A, Miljanich GP, Lambert EH. Calcium-channel antibodies in the Lambert-Eaton syndrome and other paraneoplastic syndromes. N Engl J Med 1995;332: 1467–1474.
2. Dau PC, Denys EH. Plasmapheresis and immunosuppressive drug therapy in the Eaton-Lambert syndrome. Ann Neurol 1982;11:570–575.
3. Ciavarella D, Wuest D, Strauss RG, Gilcher RO, Kasprisin DO, Kiprov DD, Klein HG, McLeod BC. Management of neurologic disorders. J Clin Apheresis 1993;8:242–257.
4. Thornton CA, Griggs RC. Plasma exchange and intravenous immunoglobulin treatment of neuromuscular disease. Ann Neurol 1994;35:260–268.
5. Assessment of plasmapheresis. Report of the Therapeutics and Technology Assessment Subcommittee of the American Academy of Neurology. Neurology 1996;47:840–843.

STIFF-MAN SYNDROME

The stiff-man syndrome is a disorder with progressive rigidity, painful spasms of limb or trunk muscles, and continuous motor unit activity (1). Vicari et al (2) described a patient with stiff-man syndrome found to have autoantibodies against glutamic acid decarboxylase (GAD). **Five 2-liter TPE treatments performed over a 12-day period were associated with a decrease in the anti-GAD titers and a disappearance of muscular rigidity (1).**

Given the paucity of available data, a recent assessment by the American Academy of Neurology concluded that TPE must be considered an investigational treatment for this disorder (3).

REFERENCES

1. Brashear HR, Phillips LH. Autoantibodies to GABAergic neurons and response to plasmapheresis in stiff man syndrome. Neurology 1991;41:1588–1592.
2. Vicari AM, Folli F, Pozza G, et al. Plasmapheresis in the treatment of stiff man syndrome. N Engl J Med 1989;320:1499. Letter.
3. Assessment of plasmapheresis. Report of the Therapeutics and Technology Assessment Subcommittee of the American Academy of Neurology. Neurology 1996;47:840–843.

AMYOTROPHIC LATERAL SCLEROSIS

A recent review of the available data regarding TPE and ALS concluded that several controlled trials, with and without immunosuppression, have not demonstrated any therapeutic benefit in the treatment of ALS (1). However, in several trials, the TPE prescription was clearly inadequate (0.5-liter exchanges), and a recent report of serum antibodies to calcium channels in patients with ALS may spark new, more adequate TPE trials (2).

Citing a previous review by an NIH Consensus Conference from 1986 (3), a recent assessment by the American Adacemy of Neurology concluded that there was no evidence that TPE had any role in the treatment of ALS (4).

REFERENCES

1. Ciavarella D, Wuest D, Strauss RG, Gilcher RO, Kasprisin DO, Kiprov DD, Klein HG, McLeod BC. Management of neurologic disorders. J Clin Apheresis 1993;8:242–257.
2. Smith RG, Hamilton S, Hofmann F, Schneider T, Nastainczyk W, Birnbaumer L, Stefani E, Appel SH. Serum antibodies to L-type calcium channels in patients with amyotrophic lateral sclerosis. N Engl J Med 1992;327:1721–1782.
3. NIH Consensus Conference. The utility of therapeutic plasmapheresis for neurological disorders. JAMA 1986;256:1333–1337.
4. Assessment of plasmapheresis. Report of the Therapeutics and

Technology Assessment Subcommittee of the American Academy of Neurology. Neurology 1996;47:840–843.

NEUROMYOTONIA (ISAACS' SYNDROME)

Neuromyotonia is a rare disorder, with suspected autoimmune etiology, in which hyperexcitability of peripheral motor nerves is associated with incapacitating muscle twitching, cramps, and weakness. **Two series of TPE treatments consisting of 10 and 5 daily treatments were performed 6 months apart and were associated with an almost complete disappearance of symptoms for a 2- to 3-week period (1).**

Considering the paucity of data, the American Academy of Neurology has concluded that TPE must be considered an investigational therapy for neuromyotonia (2).

REFERENCES

1. Sinha S, Newsom-Davis J, Mills K, Byrne N, Lang B, Vincent A. Autoimmune aetiology for acquired neuromyotonia (Isaacs' syndrome). Lancet 1991;338:75–77.
2. Assessment of plasmapheresis. Report of the Therapeutics and Technology Assessment Subcommittee of the American Academy of Neurology. Neurology 1996;47:840–843.

ACUTE DISSEMINATED ENCEPHALOMYELITIS

ADEM is a demyelinating disorder of the CNS that is thought to be immune mediated. The common presentation is that of focal neurologic deficits after a viral prodrome. A recent report by Kanter et al (1) described two well-documented cases of steroid-resistant fulminant ADEM responsive to TPE. **Successful TPE prescription involved five daily one-plasma volume exchanges in one patient and two series of six and three treatments in another patient.** In consideration of this report, an assessment by the American Academy of Neurology concluded that TPE "may be of use" in the treatment of ADEM (2).

REFERENCES

1. Kanter DS, Horensky D, Sperling RA, Kaplan JD, Malachowski ME, Churchill WH Jr. Plasmapheresis in fulminant acute disseminated encephalomyelitis. Neurology 1995;45:824–827.

2. Assessment of plasmapheresis. Report of the Therapeutics and Technology Assessment Subcommittee of the American Academy of Neurology. Neurology 1996;47:840–843.

SENSORINEURAL HEARING LOSS: IMMUNE-MEDIATED INNER EAR DISEASE

There is evidence that some patients with sensorineural hearing loss (SNHL) may have an immune-mediated disease. A common clinical profile for this entity has been defined by Hughes et al (1) and involves a middle-aged patient (often female) with bilateral, asymmetric, progressive sensorineural hearing loss, with or without dizziness, and occasional systemic immune disease such as rheumatoid arthritis. It is suggested that in this setting, immune laboratory tests (lymphocyte transformation with inner ear proteins) should be obtained and a trial of immunotherapy offered. If test results are positive and there is a beneficial response to therapy, a presumptive diagnosis of immune-mediated inner ear disease (IMIED) can be made. Barna and Hughes (2) reviewed the evidence for an immune-based pathogenesis for this entity. Amid the evidence cited in their review, most convincing is that in animal models, inner ear damage can occur after immunization with inner ear tissue and appears to be transferable with sensitized T cells. In humans, SNHL can occur in the context of systemic immunologic disease and in some cases the hearing loss can be improved by immunosuppressive therapy. These authors also provided arguments to suggest that the disease may not fit criteria for an "autoimmune" disease and that clinical inner ear disease with evidence of immunologic involvement should be termed "immune-mediated" rather than "autoimmune."

Given the clinical response with immunosuppressive therapy, Luetje (3) used TPE as a means of decreasing the need for steroid and cytotoxic medications. Improved auditory function occurred in six of eight patients. After up to 3 years of follow-up, three of six no longer required immunosuppressant medication. He concluded that TPE can stabilize or improve auditory and vestibular symptoms in certain patients with IMIED. He also suggested that TPE should be considered as a possible first-line therapy followed by cytotoxic immunosuppressants. In a subsequent report with a mean follow-up of 6.7 years, Luetje and Berliner (4) reported on 16 patients (5 men, 11 women) who underwent TPE at one or more times during the active phase of their disease. Of these, eight (50%)

had improved or stable hearing in one or both ears and only 25% of patients required continued use of immunosuppressive drugs.

In the above report, successful **TPE prescription involved a series of three treatments on alternate days. Each exchange equaled one plasma volume (3 liters) replaced with 5% albumin**. In some patients, a second series of treatments was performed later in the course of their disease.

REFERENCES

1. Hughes GB, Barna BP, Kinney SE, Calabrese LH, Nalepa NJ. Clinical diagnosis of immune inner-ear disease. Laryngoscope 1988;98:251–253.
2. Barna BP, Hughes GB. Autoimmune inner ear disease—a real entity? Clin Lab Med 1997;17:581–594.
3. Luetje CM. Theoretical and practical implications for plasmapheresis in autoimmune inner ear disease. Laryngoscope 1989;99:1137–1146.
4. Luetje CM, Berliner KI. Plasmapheresis in autoimmune inner ear disease: long-term follow-up. Am J Otol 1997;18:572–576.

REFSUM'S DISEASE

Refsum's disease is an autosomal recessive disorder associated with elevated levels of phytanic acid and is due to an enzyme deficiency in alpha oxidation. Clinical symptomatology includes retinitis pigmentosa, peripheral neuropathy, ataxia, icthyosis-like skin lesions, and cardiac arrhythmias. There is also a modest amount of renal dysfunction with proteinuria, lipiduria, declines in glomerular filtration rate and renal blood flow, and both proximal and distal tubular dysfunction (1). Phytanic acid is not endogenously produced, and its level can be limited by specialized diets. It is transported in the serum bound to lipoprotein and is removable by TPE. Several reports documented substantial clinical improvement in neuropathic and muscular disability as a result of TPE treatments (2,3). The renal functional abnormalities may also improve (1). Decreases in visual acuity do not improve. Prescription of TPE is variable and depends on the severity of the disease and the associated phytanic acid content of the recommended diet. Gibberd et al (2) calculated that TPE treatments could be performed as seldom as two times per year to remove the phytanic acid that had accumulated from a relatively restricted diet. Moser et al (3) prescribed over 100 biweekly treatments to obtain significant clinical improvement in a patient with established neurologic disability. In one series, despite a restrictive diet, 5 of 22 patients required TPE treatments. Four patients had immediate cessation of cardiac arrhythmias, whereas icthyosis, ataxia, and sensorimotor neuropathy improved more slowly (4). Normal levels of phytanic acid are below 33 μmol/L, and Gibberd (4) recommends TPE when levels exceed 1500 μmol/L. **In symptomatic patients, exchanges should be performed from twice a week to twice a month, with the goal of lowering phytanic acid levels toward normal. Maintenance TPE treatments may be monthly or as few as twice a year (5).**

Until there is an enzyme replacement therapy, TPE remains an effective option for the management of these patients. Considering the apparent irreversibility of the visual deficits, it would appear prudent to initiate some form of dietary restriction and extracorporeal removal as soon as the diagnosis is confirmed.

Because phytanic acid is transported on large-molecular-weight lipoproteins, cascade filtration, using two filters of differing sieving coefficients (see Selective Removal Techniques, Chap. 3), allows an efficient net removal while limiting the concurrent loss of albumin and immunoglobulins (6,7). Unfortunately, the secondary filters required for this type of double filtration are becoming increasingly difficult to find in the United States.

A recent assessment by the American Academy of Neurology concluded that TPE "may have a role" in lowering the levels of phytanic acid but that the role of TPE in relation to dietary restriction of phytanic acid remains to be elucidated. The Academy further concluded that TPE must be considered as an investigational treatment for Refsum's disease (8).

REFERENCES

1. Pabico RC, Gruebel BJ, McKenna BA, Griggs RC, Hollander J, Nusbacher J, Panner BJ. Renal involvement in Refsum's disease. Am J Med 1981;70:1136–1143.
2. Gibberd FB, Billimoria JD, Page NGR, Retsas S. Heredopathia atactica polyneuritiformis (Refsum's disease) treated by diet and plasma exchange. Lancet 1979;1:575–578.
3. Moser HW, Braine H, Pyeritz RE, Ullman D, Murray C, Asbury AK. Therapeutic trial of plasmapheresis in Refsum disease and Fabry disease. Birth Defects 1980;16:491–497.

4. Gibberd FB. Plasma exchange for Refsum's disease. Transfus Sci 1993;14:23–26.
5. Kasprisin DO, Strauss RG, Ciavarella D, Gilcher RO, Kiprov DD, Klein HG, McLeod BC. Management of metabolic and miscellaneous disorders. J Clin Apheresis 1993;8:231–241.
6. Siegmund JB, Meier H, Hoppmann I, Gutsche HU. Cascade filtration in Refsum's disease. Nephrol Dial Transplant 1995;10:117–119.
7. Gutsche HU, Siegmund JB, Hoppmann I. Lipapheresis: an immunoglobulin-sparing treatment for Refsum's disease. Acta Neurol Scand 1996;94:190–193.
8. Assessment of plasmapheresis. Report of the Therapeutics and Technology Assessment Subcommittee of the American Academy of Neurology. Neurology 1996;47:840–843.

Hematologic Disorders

8

Hyperviscosity Syndrome   110
Cryoglobulinemia   114
Thrombotic Thrombocytopenic Purpura   118
    TTP in Pregnancy   122
    HELLP Syndrome   123
    HUS in Adults   125
    HUS in Children   128
Idiopathic Thrombocytopenic Purpura   129
Post-Transfusion Purpura   133
Autoimmune Hemolytic Anemia   134
    Cold Agglutinins   134
    Warm Agglutinins   134
Maternal-Fetal Incompatibility: Rh Disease   136
Hemophilia: Removal of Factor VIII Inhibitors   137

Because the indication for therapeutic plasma exchange (TPE) in multiple myeloma is related to renal failure, this disorder is reviewed in Chapter 12. Macroglobulinemic- and cryoglobulinemic-associated polyneuropathies are discussed in Chapter 7. The remaining indications for TPE in hematologic diseases are listed and rated in Table 8-1.

HYPERVISCOSITY SYNDROME

The hyperviscosity syndrome results from the presence in serum of high levels of proteins capable of increasing the serum viscosity as measured by an Ostwald viscosimeter. Classically, the syndrome is a result of increased amounts of IgM, as seen in Waldenström's macroglobulinemia, but abnormal polymers of IgA, IgG, and kappa

Table 8-1. Hematologic Indications for TPE

	References and Year		
	1 **1986**	**2** **1993**	**3** **1994**
		Rating	
Hematologic disorders			
Hyperviscosity syndrome	I	I	I
Cryoglobulinemia	II	I	I
TTP/HUS	I	I	I
HELLP syndrome	nl	II	II
ITP	III	III	III
Post-transfusion purpura	II	I	I
Autoimmune hemolytic anemia	III	III	III
Maternal-fetal incompatibility Rh disease	II	III	nl
Removal of factor VIII inhibitors	II	II	III

Rating: I, standard therapy, acceptable but not mandatory; II, available evidence tends to favor efficacy: conventional therapy usually tried first; III, inadequately tested at this time; IV, no demonstrated value in controlled trials. nl, not listed.

REFERENCES: 1. American Medical Association Council on Scientific Affairs. Current status of therapeutic plasmapheresis. JAMA 1985;253:819–825.

2. Strauss RG, Ciavarella D, Gilcher RO, Kasprisin DO, Kiprov DD, Klein HG, McLeod BC. An overview of current management. J Clin Apheresis 1993;8:189–194.

3. Leitman SF, Ciavarella D, McLeod B, Owen H, Price T, Sniecinski I. Guidelines for therapeutic hemapheresis. Bethesda, MD: American Association of Blood Banks, revised 1994.

light chains have also been implicated in certain cases of multiple myeloma (1–3). Clinical signs result from impaired microcirculation in the brain, digits, kidneys, eye, and peripheral nerves (see Paraprotein-Associated Polyneuropathy, Chap. 7). Acute symptomatology includes headache, dizziness, vertigo, nystagmus, hearing loss, visual impairment, somnolence, coma, and seizures. Mucosal hemorrhage may result from impaired platelet function, and signs of congestive heart failure have been attributed to an expanded plasma volume. Sausage-like beeding of the retinal veins is a classic clinical sign. The diagnosis is made by the documentation of an increased serum viscosity. Normal serum viscosity is between 1.4 and 1.8 (measured as the flow time of serum divided by that of water). **Patients with values between 2 and 4 are only rarely symptomatic, but most patients with values between 5 and 8 are affected (1). With values above 10, all patients are**

symptomatic. Corresponding values for IgM are commonly between 4 and 8 g/dL, but correlation with viscosity values is not linear (4). Total serum protein levels are usually 10 g/dL or more.

Plasma exchange is universally accepted as effective treatment for acute symptomatology (1,4–7) and, on occasion, can yield dramatic results (reversal of coma during the treatment [5]). Those presenting with severe neurologic impairment, such as stupor or coma, should be treated on an emergency basis. The number and timing of the TPE treatments are dependent on the initial viscosity values and the implicated proteins (i.e., IgM versus IgA or IgG polymers). **A reasonable initial prescription would be a one plasma volume exchange (see below), replaced with albumin, repeated daily until symptoms subside or until serum viscosity is returned to normal**. Treating IgM-related hyperviscosity, **Solomon and Fahey (4) described acute management requiring between 5 and 20 liters of exchanged plasma**. IgM-related syndromes respond most quickly because 80% of these proteins are intravascular (8). IgA- or IgG-related syndromes may require a greater volume and a more repetitive treatment schedule, because most of these immunoglobulins are extravascular and successful lowering of serum values is followed by extravascular to intravascular redistribution (9,10). Of further note is that hyperviscosity syndromes are likely to increase the plasma volume beyond that calculated by commonly used formulas (1,11). As an example, using isotopically labeled albumin, we documented a 6.7-liter plasma volume in a patient in which the calculated value was only 4 liters (12). Technically, albumin replacement requirements can be reduced or eliminated by cascade filtration using secondary filters capable of concentrating very large-molecular-weight proteins while allowing albumin to be returned to the patient (13). Despite the need for less replacement fluid, cascade filtration may be substantially less efficient, and a recent comparison study demonstrated a 48% reduction in plasma viscosity for standard TPE and only a 26% reduction with cascade filtration (14). In any event, the secondary filters required for cascade filtration are becoming increasingly difficult to obtain in the United States.

Most symptoms will reverse with successful lowering of serum viscosity, but persistent hearing loss has been described and attributed to venous thrombosis of the inner ear (1). Peripheral neuropathy may take longer to reverse (15) (see Paraprotein-Associated Polyneuropathy, Chap. 7). Because plasmapheresis does not affect the disease process, cessation of plasma exchange treatments, in the absence of other therapy, results in a recurrence of symptoms within 2 to 3 weeks (1). Chemotherapy with chlorambucil and cyclophosphamide has been used for chronic management. A recent report describes treatment of Waldenström's macroglobulinemia with 2-chlorodeoxyadenosine (16).

REFERENCES

1. Bloch KJ, Maki DG. Hyperviscosity syndromes associated with immunoglobulin abnormalities. Semin Hematol 1973;10:113–124.
2. Carter PW, Cohen HJ, Crawford J. Hyperviscosity syndrome in association with kappa light chain myeloma. Am J Med 1989;86:591–601.
3. Bachrach HJ, Myers JB, Bartholomew WR. A unique case of kappa light chain disease associated with cryoglobulinemia, pyroglobulinemia and hyperviscosity syndrome. Am J Med 1989;86:596–602.
4. Solomon A, Fahey JL. Plasmapheresis therapy in macroglobulinemia. Ann Intern Med 1963;58:789–800.
5. Isbister JP, Biggs JC, Penny R. Experience with large volume plasmapheresis in malignant paraproteinemia and immune disorders. Aust N Z J Med 1978;8:154–164.
6. American Medical Association Council on Scientific Affairs. Current status of therapeutic plasmapheresis. JAMA 1985;253:819–825.
7. Gilcher RO, Strauss RG, Ciavarella D, Kasprisin DO, Kiprov DD, Klein HG, McLeod BC. Management of renal disorders. J Clin Apheresis 1993;8:258–269.
8. Barth WF, Wochner D, Waldmann TA, Fahey JL. Metabolism of human gamma macroglobulins. J Clin Invest 1964;43:1036–1048.
9. Cohen S, Freeman T. Metabolic heterogeneity of human gamma globulin. Biochem J 1960;76:475–487.
10. Kaplan AA. Towards a rational prescription of plasma exchange: the kinetics of immunoglobulin removal. Semin Dial 1992;5:227–229.
11. Alexanian R. Blood volume in monoclonal gammopathy. Blood 1977;49:301–306.
12. Kaplan AA, Halley SE. Plasma exchange with a rotating filter. Kidney Int 1990;38:160–166.

13. Valbonesi M, Mosconi L, Montani F, Florio G, Rossi U. Cascade filtration: clinical application in 26 patients with immune complex and IgM mediated diseases. Int J Artif Organs 1983;6:303–307.
14. Hoffkes HG, Heemann UW, Teschendorf C, Uppenkamp M, Philipp T. Hyperviscosity syndrome: efficacy and comparison of plasma exchange by plasma separation and cascade filtration in patients with immunocytoma of Waldenström's type. Clin Nephrol 1995;43:335–338.
15. Dellagi K, Dupouey P, Brouet JC, Billecocq A, Gomez D, Clauvel JP, Seligmann M. Waldenström's macroglobulinemia and peripheral neuropathy: a clinical and immunologic study. Blood 1983;62:280–285.
16. Dmopoulos MA, Kantarjian H, Estey E, O'Brein S, et al. Treatment of Waldenström's macroglobulinemia with 2-chlorodeoxyadenosine. Ann Intern Med 1993;118:193–198.

CRYOGLOBULINEMIA

Cryoglobulins are immunoglobulins or immunoglobulin-containing complexes that reversibly precipitate on exposure to cold and redissolve on warming. Three general types have been described: type I, which is comprised of monoclonal proteins and associated with disorders such as myeloma, Waldenström's macroglobulinemia, and other lymphoproliferative disorders; type II, which is comprised of mixed cryoglobulins with a monoclonal component and is associated with lymphoproliferative disorders, autoimmune diseases, and viral infections; and type III, comprised of mixed cryoglobulins with polyclonal components and is associated with hepatitis C infection (1). Type I cryoglobulins are often associated with impaired blood flow with symptoms of Raynaud's phenomenon, acrocyanosis, purpura, and gangrene of fingers and toes. Renal disease may be associated with cryoglobulin deposition in the glomerular capillaries (2). Types II and III often present as immune-complex-mediated diseases with complement activation and vasculitis. Mixed "essential" cryoglobulinemia may present with palpable purpura, lymphadenopathy, hepatosplenomegaly, peripheral neuropathy, and glomerulonephritis.

There has never been a randomized controlled study of plasmapheresis for cryoglobulinemia. Nonetheless, the clearcut rationale for its use (the removal of the pathogenic cryoglobulins), numerous successful case reports, uncontrolled studies, and the opinion of the most experienced investigators have led to a general consensus that TPE is a useful adjunct for the treatment of severe active disease as manifested by progressive renal failure, coalescing purpura, or advanced neuropathy (1–10). There has also been successful experience in the use of TPE for the chronic management of cryoglobulinemia, with one patient receiving 238 treatments over a 12-year period (11), but current indications for this approach are less clear, especially with the recent reports of successful management of hepatitis C–associated disease with interferon (12).

In general, TPE is performed in conjunction with the administration of steroids and immunosuppressive agents, but the recent implication of hepatitis C viral infection as an etiologic factor in many patients with mixed "essential" cryoglobulinemia (13) is worrisome and suggests that immunosuppressive agents may be detrimental. Indeed, in our own limited experience, we witnessed the rapid resolution of nephritic renal failure and severe purpuric lesions with TPE alone, without the concomitant use of steroids or immunosuppressive agents. Similarly, Ferri et al (9) reported on four patients whose renal disease was successfully managed with TPE alone without steroids or cytotoxic agents.

A reasonable plasmapheresis prescription is to exchange one plasma volume three times weekly for 2 to 3 weeks. In one successful series of 15 patients, D'Amico et al (17) reported that **an average of 13 treatments were required to induce clinical improvement (range, 4 to 39)**. Frankel et al (11) prescribed 3 to 12 daily exchanges for their initial approach. The **replacement fluid** can be 5% albumin, which **must be warmed to prevent precipitation of circulating cryoglobulins** (8,11). An associated peripheral neuropathy may be vasculitic in nature and may require a greater time for reversal of symptoms (see Paraprotein-Associated Polyneuropathy, Chap. 7).

Selective removal techniques can be used to eliminate or minimize the need for replacement fluid. Double cascade filtration uses a "secondary" filter that allows the removed plasma to be separated into relatively small (albumin, IgG, etc.) and relatively large proteins (the multimeric cryoglobulins) with the smaller protein fraction being reinfused to the patient and the larger protein fraction being discarded. Although this is an elegant technique that can substantially reduce the need for replacement fluid, the two–step filtration process is more time-consuming and the secondary filter is expensive, prone to clotting, and is becoming difficult to obtain in the United States (14). Cryofiltration selectively removes the circulating cryoglobulins by cooling the plasma in an extracorporeal circuit, but the technique is most efficiently performed by a continuous online process requiring a specialized machine designed for this purpose (15). Alternatively, one can perform a two-step procedure where the patient's own plasma can be reinfused after incubation in the cold to precipitate out the abnormal proteins (16).

The optimal method for assessing the efficacy of plasmapheresis is uncertain. In certain cases, there may be dramatic clinical improvement with a rapid reversal of purpura (after two or three treatments) or a substantial improvement in renal function after a recent elevation in serum creatinine. Neuropathy, however, is unlikely to respond during short-term therapy, and it becomes desirable to follow an objective serologic parameter to guide the need for additional treatments (17,18). Changes in the percent cryocrit after plasmapheresis do not correlate closely with clinical activity because this test is performed at such a low temperature that even small amounts of cryoprotein may result in detectable precipitation. It has been suggested that the percent solubility of the cryoglobulins at 37°C or a decline in the temperature at which the cryoproteins precipitate may be a better index of the response to therapy (4,19), but these tests are not commonly performed.

There is evidence that interferon alfa can lead to a reduction in circulating cryoglobulin levels and clinical remission (12). Unfortunately, disease activity can recur after discontinuation of interferon. Considering the delayed onset of clinical response to the reinitiation of interferon, TPE can be useful as the initial immediate therapy for these exacerbations. If standard plasma exchange is used (as opposed to the selective techniques described above) and interferon therapy is initiated during a series of plasma exchange treatments, it should be administered immediately after the treatment to minimize its removal.

REFERENCES

1. Malchesky PS, Clough JD. Cryoglobulins: properties, prevalence in disease and removal. Cleve Clin Q 1985;52:175–192.
2. Gilcher RO, Strauss RG, Ciavarella D, Kasprisin DO, Kiprov DD, Klein HG, McLeod BC. Management of renal disorders. J Clin Apheresis 1993;8:258–269.
3. Solomon A, Fahey JL. Plasmapheresis therapy in macroglobulinemia. Ann Intern Med 1963;58:789–800.

4. Lockwood CM. Lymphoma, cryoglobulinemia and renal disease. Kidney Int 1979;16:522–530.
5. Berkman EM, Orlin JB. Use of plasmapheresis and partial plasma exchange in the management of patients with cryoglobulinemia. Transfusion 1979;20:171–178.
6. Geltner D, Kohn RW, Gorevic P, Franklin EC. The effect of combination therapy (steroids, immunosuppressives and plasmapheresis) on 5 mixed cryoglobulinemia patients with renal, neurologic and vascular involvement. Arthritis Rheum 1981; 24:1121–1127.
7. D'Amico G, Ferrario F, Colasanti G, Bucci A. Glomerulonephritis in essential mixed cryoglobulinemia. In: Davison PJ, Guillon PJ, eds. Proceedings of the XXI Congress of the European Dialysis and Transplant Association. London: Pitman, 1984:527–548.
8. Evans TW, Nicholls AJ, Shortland JR, Ward AM, Brown CB. Acute renal failure in essential mixed cryoglobulinemia: precipitation and reversal by plasma exchange. Clin Nephrol 1984;21:287–293.
9. Ferri C, Moriconi L, Gremignai G, Migliorini P, Paleologo G, Fosellar PV, Bombardieri S. Treatment of the renal involvement in mixed cryoglobulinemia with prolonged plasma exchange. Nephron 1986;42:246–253.
10. D'Amico G, Colasanti G, Ferrario F, Sinico RA. Renal involvement in essential mixed cryoglobulinemia. Kidney Int 1989;35: 1004–1014.
11. Frankel AH, Singer DRJ, Winearls CG, Evans DJ, Rees AJ, Pusey CD. Type II essential mixed cryoglobulinemia: presentation, treatment and outcome in 13 patients. Q J Med 1992;82:101–124.
12. Misiani R, Bellavita P, Fenili D, Vicari O, Marchesi D, Sironi PL, Zilio P, Vernocchi A, Massazza M, Vendramin G, Tfanzi E, Zanetti A. Interferon alfa-2a therapy in cryoglobulinemia associated with hepatitis C virus. N Engl J Med 1994;330: 751–756.
13. Misiani R, Bellavita P, Fenili D, Borelli G, Marchesi D, Massazza M, Vendramin G, Comotti B, Tanzi F, Scudeller G, Zanetti A. Hepatitis C virus infection in patients with essential mixed cryoglobulinemia. Ann Intern Med 1992;117: 573–577.
14. Valbonesi M, Garelli S, Montani F, Cefis M, Rossi U. Management of immune-mediated and paraproteinemic diseases by

membrane plasma separation and cascade filtration. Vox Sang 1982;43:91–101.

15. Vibert GJ, Wirtz SA, Smith JW, et al. Cryofiltration as an alternative to plasma exchange: plasma macromolecular solute removal without replacement fluids. In: Nose Y, Malchesky PS, Smith JW, eds. Plasmapheresis. Cleveland: ISAO Press, 1983:281–287.

16. McLeod BC, Sassetti RJ. Plasmapheresis with return of cryoglobulin-depleted autologous plasma (cryoglobulinpheresis) in cryoglobulinemia. Blood 1980;55:866–870.

17. Chad D, Oaruser JM, Bradley WG, Adelman LS, Pinn VW. The pathogenesis of cryoglobulinemic neuropathy. Neurology 1982;32:725–729.

18. Berkman EM, Orlin JB. Use of plasmapheresis and partial plasma exchange in the management of patients with cryo-globulinemia. Transfusion 1980;20:171–178.

19. Valbonesi M, Mosconi L, Montani F, Florio G, Rossi U. A method for the study of cryoglobulin solubilization curves at 37 degrees Celsius. Preliminary studies and application to plasma exchange in cryoglobulinemic syndromes. Int J Artif Organs 1983;6:87–90.

THROMBOTIC THROMBOCYTOPENIC PURPURA

Thrombotic thrombocytopenic purpura (TTP) is a syndrome characterized by thrombocytopenia, microangiopathic hemolytic anemia, neurologic abnormalities, fever, and renal dysfunction. Although there has been varied treatment success with corticosteroids, antiplatelet agents, and splenectomy (1,2), there is currently a general agreement in the literature that plasma exchange with replacement by fresh frozen plasma (FFP) or cryosupernatant (see below) is the treatment of choice (3–7). Prior to the use of plasmapheresis, mortality with TTP was as high as 90% (8).

The pathogenesis of the microthrombotic lesions of TTP is only incompletely understood. One hypothesis suggests that an unknown toxin promotes the endothelial release of particularly large multimers of von Willebrand (vW) factor that in turn promote platelet aggregation. The same toxin may also promote the release of a platelet-activating factor. Alternatively, or concurrently, a toxic stimulus may change the normal anticoagulant phenotype of the endothelium. There is also evidence that the plasma may lack endothelial-derived anticoagulant or fibrinolytic factors such as tissue plasminogen activator, thrombomodulin, or prostacyclin (9–12). It is therefore unclear whether the major factor in the pathogenic platelet aggregation is either the presence of a procoagulant factor or the absence of an antithrombotic factor. As a result, controversy remains whether treatment should be aimed at removing the procoagulant(s) or replacing the antithrombotic factor(s). Translating this controversy to currently available treatment options, it is still unresolved whether plasma exchange or plasma infusion is the best treatment for TTP.

In the largest controlled trial of its type, 102 patients were randomized to receive either plasma exchange with FFP or plasma infusion alone (the Canadian Apheresis Group) (Table 8-2) (13). All patients also received aspirin and dipyridamole. Because plasma infusion alone was limited by the onset of intravascular volume overload, the patients receiving plasma exchange received three

Table 8-2.   Controlled Trial of TPE vs. Plasma Infusion for TTP

	TPE	Plasma Infusion	
Baseline			
Number of patients	51	51	
Platelets ($\times 10^{-9}$/L)	22.4	24.1	
Hematocrit	0.26	0.25	
Lactate dehydrogenase (U/L)	1407	1248	
Results after 9 days of treatment			
Success[a]	24 (47%)	13 (25%)	
Failure[a]	27 (53%)	38 (75%)	
Survived	49 (96%)	43 (84%)	
Died	2 (4%)	8 (16%)	
Results after 6 months		*no TPE*	*with TPE[b]*
Number of patients	51	32	19
Success[a]	40 (78%)[a]	10 (31%)	15 (79%)
Failure[a]	11 (22%)[a]	22 (69%)	4 (21%)
Overall survival			
Number of patients	51	20	31
Survived	40 (78%)	10 (50%)	22 (71%)
Died	11 (22%)	10 (50%)	9 (29%)

[a] $p < 0.025$ between groups.
[b] Patients who failed plasma infusion after 9 days were offered TPE.
SOURCE: Adapted from Rock GA, Shumak KH, Buskand NA, et al. Comparison of plasma exchange with plasma infusion in the treatment of thrombotic thrombocytopenic purpura. N Engl J Med 1991;325:393.

119

times the amount of plasma. At 6 months, the remission rate and survival rate were statistically higher in the group receiving plasma exchange (78% versus 31% remission and 78% versus 50% for survival). Thus, despite the clear superior results in the TPE group, it is sobering to note that there remains a 22% mortality in the group treated with plasma exchange and a 50% mortality in those receiving plasma infusion alone, underscoring the significant lethality of this disease.

Unfortunately, the results of the above-mentioned trial do not answer the question of whether plasma exchange is more beneficial than plasma infusion alone, because the plasma exchange group received three times more plasma than the infusion group. Keeping the controversy alive, one recent report described a patient with relapsing TTP in which plasma infusion, either alone or as part of plasma exchange, led to remission of the disease, whereas plasma exchange with saline or albumin was ineffective on three different occasions (14).

In general, **plasma exchange *with FFP replacement* is performed daily until the platelet count is normalized and hemolysis has largely ceased** (as evident in part by a lactate dehydrogenase [LDH] level below 400 and the disappearance of schistocytes on the peripheral blood smear). On average, **7 to 16 daily exchanges (range, 3 to 107) are required to induce remission** (2,13). The recommended **volume to be exchanged is 1.5 times the estimated plasma volume for the first three treatments followed by one plasma volume exchanges thereafter** (13). Despite the documented success with FFP, it has been suggested that the infusion of large amounts of vW factor in the FFP may promote further platelet aggregation. Thus, in patients resistant to TPE treatments, the use of cryosupernatant may be preferable because vW factor is largely removed in the cryoprecipitate (15).

In those patients responding to plasma exchange, Rock et al (13) reported an early relapse in 10 patients (~40%) with decreases in platelet counts occurring in a mean of 5 days. On average, these patients required an additional 15 exchanges over the following 20 days to achieve a complete response. Bell et al (2) reported a relapse rate as high as 86%, occurring within 30 to 60 days, but their treatment regimen was less aggressive and included corticosteroids. Late relapses, occurring between 3 and 10 years, were reported as a follow-up to the Canadian Apheresis Group trial, revealing that more than one-third of patients who survived the original episode had at least one relapse within 10 years (16).

TTP is the only disease treated with plasmapheresis for which **FFP (or cryosupernatant) is the required replacement fluid**. Large volumes of FFP (~4–5 U/L of plasma removed) from many different donors are required, increasing the risk of anaphylactoid reactions. Patients with severe and repetitive reactions to FFP can be pretreated with ephedrine, prednisone, and diphenhydramine (17). Our own protocol prescribes oral doses of 50 mg of prednisone given 13, 7, and 1 hour before the treatment, combined with 50 mg of diphenhydramine and 25 mg of ephedrine given 1 hour before treatment. **In the event of a severe life-threatening reaction (laryngeal edema, etc.), 0.3–0.5 mL of epinephrine should be available for subcutaneous administration.**

REFERENCES

1. Cuttner J. Thrombotic thrombocytopenic purpura: a ten year experience. Blood 1980;56:302–306.
2. Bell WR, Braine HG, Ness PM, Kickler TS. Improved survival of thrombotic thrombocytopenic purpura-hemolytic uremic syndrome: clinical experience in 108 patients. N Engl J Med 1991;325:398–403.
3. Brekenridge RL Jr, Solberg LS, Pineda AA, Petitt RM, Dharkar DD. Treatment of thrombotic thrombocytopenic purpura with plasma exchange, antiplatelet agents, corticosteroid and plasma infusion: Mayo Clinic experience. J Clin Apheresis 1982;1: 6–13.
4. Henon P. Treatment of thrombotic thrombocytopenic purpura. First results of a controlled clinical trial. Plasma Ther Transfus Technol 1986;7:101–106.
5. Onundarson PT, Rowe JM, Heal JM, Francis CW. Response to plasma exchange and splenectomy in thrombotic thrombocytopenic purpura: a 10 year experience at a single institution. Arch Intern Med 1992;152:791–796.
6. Moake JL. TTP-desperation, empiricism, progress. N Engl J Med 1991;325:426–428. Editorial.
7. Gilcher RO, Strauss RG, Ciavarella D, Kasprisin DO, Kiprov DD, Klein HG, McLeod BC. Management of renal disorders. J Clin Apheresis 1993;8:258–269.

8. Amorosi EL, Ultman JE. Thrombotic thrombocytopenic purpura: report of 16 cases and review of the literature. Medicine 1966;45:139–159.
9. Byrnes JJ, Moake JL. Thrombotic thrombocytopenic purpura and the haemolytic uraemic syndrome: evolving concepts of pathogenesis and therapy. Clin Haematol 1986;15:413–442.
10. Kwaan HC. Clinicopathologic features of thrombotic thrombocytopenic purpura. Semin Hematol 1987;24:71–81.
11. Lian EC-Y. Pathogenesis of thrombotic thrombocytopenic purpura. Semin Hematol 1987;24:82–100.
12. Remuzzi G. HUS and TTP: variable expression of a single entity. Kidney Int 1987;32:292–308.
13. Rock GA, Shumak KH, Buskard NA, Blanchette VS, Kelton JG, Nair RC, Spasoff RA. Comparison of plasma exchange with plasma infusion in the treatment of thrombotic thrombocytopenic purpura. N Engl J Med 1991;325:393–397.
14. Ruggenenti P, Galbusera M, Cornejo RP, Bellavita P, Remuzzi G. Thrombotic thrombocytopenic purpura: evidence that infusion rather than removal of plasma induces remission of the disease. Am J Kidney Dis 1993;21:314–318.
15. Byrnes JJ, Moake JL, Klug P, Periman P. Effectiveness of the cryosupernatant fraction of plasma in the treatment of refractory thrombotic thrombocytopenic purpura. Ann J Hematol 1990;34:169–174.
16. Shumak KH, Rock GA, Nair RC, the Canadian Apheresis Group. Late relapses in patients successfully treated for thrombotic thrombocytopenic purpura. Ann Intern Med 1995; 122:569–572.
17. Apter AJ, Kaplan AA. An approach to immunologic reactions associated with plasma exchange. J Allergy Clin Immunol 1992;90:119–124.

TTP in Pregnancy

The differential diagnosis of thrombocytopenia in pregnancy includes TTP, hemolytic-uremic syndrome (HUS), idiopathic thrombocytopenia purpura (ITP), pre-eclampsia with HELLP syndrome (hemolysis, elevated liver enzymes, and thrombocytopenia), and Evan's syndrome (1). Distinction between TTP and HUS can be difficult, but neurologic manifestations usually predominate in TTP, whereas renal abnormalities are often more prominent in HUS (2). HELLP syndrome in conjunction with pre-eclampsia can usually be distinguished from HUS and TTP by the presence of hypertension and elevated liver-derived transaminases, whereas the hemolysis of Evan's syndrome can be distinguished by a positive Coombs' test. ITP is an isolated platelet disorder without evidence of hemolysis, which should not present a difficult diagnostic dilemma with the previously mentioned syndromes.

Considering the dismal prognosis of TTP in pregnancy before the initiation of plasma manipulations (1/27 maternal survivors after 2 years, only 7/25 fetal survivors) (3) and the clear superiority of TPE in nonpregnant patients, plasma exchange is also the treatment of choice for TTP during pregnancy (1,4). Of note is that despite the possibility of treatment-induced removal of pregnancy-maintaining hormones, TPE has been successfully used from as early as the sixth week of gestation with a positive outcome in both mother and fetus (1,5,6).

REFERENCES

1. Mokrzycki MH, Rickles FR, Kaplan AA, Kohn OF. Thrombotic thrombocytopenic purpura in pregnancy: successful treatment with plasma exchange. Blood Purif 1995;13:271–281.
2. Kwann HC. Thrombotic thrombocytopenic purpura and hemolytic uremic syndrome in pregnancy. Clin Obstet Gynecol 1985;28:101–106.
3. May HV, Harbert GM Jr, Thronton WN Jr. Thrombotic thrombocytopenic purpura associated with pregnancy. Am J Obstet Gynecol 1976;126:452–458.
4. Ambrose A, Welham RT, Cefalo RC. Thrombotic thrombocytopenic purpura in early pregnancy. Obstet Gynecol 1985; 66:267–272.
5. Gerhardt RE, Koethe JD, Ntoso KS, et al. Plasma separation in pregnancy. Am Soc Artif Intern Organs 1991;20:1. Abstract.
6. Gerhardt RE, Koethe JD, Ntoso KA, Lodge S, Schlaff S, Wolf CJ. Effects of feto-placental markers with plasma exchange in pregnancy. J Clin Apheresis 1994;9:6–9.

HELLP Syndrome

As noted above, HELLP syndrome represents one of the differential diagnoses of thrombocytopenia in pregnancy. Martin et al (1) reported their 10-year experience using TPE in the management of HELLP syndrome in the postpartum period. A total of 18 patients were treated with single or multiple TPE treatments with FFP as the replacement. Indications for treatment were divided into two groups: those who had persistent evidence of HELLP syndrome for more than 72 hours after delivery (group 1) and those with evidence of worsening HELLP syndrome in association with single- or multiple-organ injury (group 2). The nine patients in group 1 with persistent postpartum HELLP syndrome responded rapidly to one or two plasma exchange procedures with no maternal deaths. In contrast, in the nine patients of group 2, when HELLP was complicated by other organ disease, the response to plasma exchange was variable and there were two deaths. These same authors also reported on the successful use of TPE in the immediate peripartal period in two patients with severe HELLP syndrome (2). In contrast, these authors found no success in the use of TPE for patients with pre-eclampsia/eclampsia syndrome without HELLP (3).

Experience from another center also noted success in the application of TPE in four patients with postpartum HELLP syndrome (4). TPE with FFP was instituted from 1 to 7 days postpartum. An average of four treatments was needed (range, one to eight). Aspartate amino transferase (AST) was the first parameter to peak and the first to normalize. Once platelet counts attained 100×10^9/L, no additional exchanges were necessary. Laboratory values normalized in the following order: AST, hemoglobin, platelets, and LDH. The authors concluded that awaiting normal LDH levels as an indicator for cessation of plasma exchange therapy would result in many unnecessary procedures.

REFERENCES

1. Martin JN Jr, Files JC, Blake PG, Perry KG Jr, Morrison JC, Norman PH. Postpartum plasma exchange for atypical preeclampsia–eclampsia as HELLP (hemolysis, elevated liver enzymes, and low platelets) syndrome. Am J Obstet Gynecol 1995;172:1107–1125.
2. Martin JN Jr, Perry KG Jr, Roberts WE, Files JC, Norman PF, Morrison JC, Blake PG. Plasma exchange for preeclampsia. III. Immediate peripartal utilization for selected patients with HELLP syndrome. J Clin Apheresis 1994;9:162–165.
3. Martin JN Jr, Perry KG Jr, Roberts WE, Norman PF, Files JC, Blake PG, Morrison JC, Wiser WL. Plasma exchange for preeclampsia. II. Unsuccessful antepartum utilization for severe preeclampsia with or without HELLP syndrome. J Clin Apheresis 1994;9:155–161.

4. Julius CJ, Dunn ZL, Blazina JF. HELLP syndrome: laboratory parameters and clinical course in four patients treated with plasma exchange. J Clin Apheresis 1994;9:228–235.

HUS in Adults

Distinction between adult HUS and TTP can be difficult, and there are those who believe that they are variable expressions of the same entity (1). In general, however, neurologic manifestations tend to dominate the clinical picture of TTP, whereas renal failure tends to be prominent in HUS. Distinction may also be possible when a clear etiologic agent can be identified, such as the association of HUS with the verotoxin produced by *Escherichia coli* 0157-H7 (2), or by the presence of certain inciting drugs such as cyclosporine, mitomycin, cisplatin, quinine, or oral contraceptives (3–5) or associated diseases (systemic lupus erythematosus, carcinoma, etc.) (6). In contrast with HUS in children, the prognosis of HUS in the adult is poor, with an estimated mortality between 25 and 50% and an incidence of end-stage renal disease of up to 40% in the remaining survivors (6–8). A recent review combining TTP and HUS found that dialysis was required in 11 of 68 cases (9). Of these 11, 4 expired during hospitalization but 5 of the remaining 7 were able to come off dialysis after a period ranging between 4 and 120 days. The authors suggest that the poorer renal outcome in previous older studies was obtained before the general use of TPE, which was used on all of their patients. Considering the difficulty in distinguishing adult HUS from TTP and the similarity in their pathology and mortality, it would seem prudent to approach this entity in a similar fashion as with TTP, with the early and intensive initiation of plasma exchange.

Mitomycin-induced cancer-associated HUS: An exceptional situation may exist in the context of mitomycin-induced cancer-associated HUS, in which plasma perfusion over a protein A column has been reported to be more effective than standard plasma exchange (10). In an uncontrolled trial of 11 patients with this condition, protein A immunoadsorption was found to be successful in 9 patients, with a stabilization of progressive renal failure achieved in 6 of these 9 (11). The treatment consisted of the removal of a mean 400mL of plasma with perfusion of the plasma over the protein A column and its subsequent return to the patient. The number of treatments ranged from 2 to 15. Although not specifically noted in this report, it would seem that the Prosorba column from

Cypress Bioscience (San Diego, CA) would allow one to provide this therapy (see Immunoadsorbant Techniques, Chap. 3). In another report, an apparent case of cisplatin-associated HUS did not respond to four plasma exchange treatments but did respond to four 2000-mL plasma perfusions over a Prosorba column (12). In data obtained by retrospective questionnaire, Snyder et al (13) reported that plasma perfusion over the Prosorba protein A column resulted in a successful treatment for 25 of 55 patients with chemotherapy-associated HUS/TTP. Although the report purports to show a substantial benefit to immunoadsorbant therapy, four of five non-responders subsequently responded to alternate treatments involving standard TPE with FFP. Thus, with the exception of this one clearly defined situation (mitomycin- or cisplatin-induced HUS) and considering that even mitomycin- or cisplatin-induced HUS has been successfully treated with standard TPE (3,14,15), the remainder of the available literature would support the use of standard plasma exchange for the treatment of HUS (9,16,17).

Recurrent HUS in renal transplantation: Recurrent HUS in patients who have received renal transplant after losing renal function to an original episode of HUS is a well-documented problem. In the differential diagnosis of HUS in the renal transplant patient are acute vascular rejection of the allograft, cyclosporine, FK506 or antilymphocyte antibody nephrotoxicity, and malignant hypertension. In an extensive review of the literature, Agarwal et al (18) noted 19 reports describing 68 cases. They concluded that TPE remains an efficacious treatment but that end points in terminating the treatments are not well defined. Although improvement or normalization in clinical status, hematocrit, LDH, peripheral schistocytes and reticulocytes, and haptoglobin may all be used as criteria for successful treatment, it is not clear if awaiting the return of renal function should be a reasonable goal before terminating the TPE procedures.

REFERENCES

1. Remuzzi G. HUS and TTP: variable expression of a single entity. Kidney Int 1987;32:292–308.
2. Rondeau E, Peraldi MN. *Escherichia coli* and the hemolytic uremic syndrome. N Engl J Med 1996;335:660–662. Editorial.
3. Drummond KN. Hemolytic uremic syndrome—then and now. N Engl J Med 1985;312:116–118. Editorial.

4. Lyman NW, Michaelson R, Viscuso RL, Winn R, Mulgaonkar V, Jacobs MG. Mitomycin-induced hemolytic-uremic syndrome: successful treatment with corticosteroids and intense plasma exchange. Arch Intern Med 1983;143:1617–1618.

5. Aster RH. Quinine sensitivity: a new cause of the hemolytic uremic syndrome. Ann Intern Med 1993;119:243–244.

6. Melnyk AMS, Solez K, Kjellstrand CM. Adult hemolytic uremic syndrome: a review of 37 cases. Arch Intern Med 1995;155:2077–2084.

7. Morel-Maroger L, Kanfer A, Solez K, et al. Prognostic importance of vascular lesions in acute renal failure with microangiopathic hemolytic anemia (hemolytic uremic syndrome): clinicopathologic study in 20 adults. Kidney Int 1979;15: 548–558.

8. Schieppati A, Ruggenenti P, Cornejo RP, et al. Renal function at hospital admission as a prognostic factor in adult hemolytic uremic syndrome. J Am Soc Nephrol 1992;2:1640–1644.

9. Conlon PJ, Howell DN, Macik G, Kovalik EC, Smith SR. The renal manifestations and outcome of thrombotic thrombocytopenic pupura/hemolytic uremic syndrome. Nephrol Dial Transpl 1195;10:1189–1193.

10. Lesesne JB, Rothschild N, Erickson B, et al. Cancer associated hemolytic-uremic syndrome: analysis of 85 cases from a national registry. J Clin Oncol 1989;7:781.

11. Korec S, Schein PS, Smith FP, Neefe JR, Wooley PV, Goldberg RM, Phillips TM. Treatment of cancer-associated hemolytic uremic syndrome with staphylococcal protein A immunoperfusion. J Clin Oncol 1986;4:210–215.

12. Watson PR, Guthrie TH Jr, Caruana RJ. Cisplatin-associated hemolytic-uremic syndrome. Cancer 1989;64:1400–1403.

13. Snyder HJ, Mittleman A, Oral A, Messerschmidt GL, Henry DH, Korec S, Bertram JH, Guthrie TH, Ciavarella D, Wuest D, Perkins W, Balint JP, Cochran SK, Peugeot RL, Jones FR. Treatment of cancer chemotherapy-associated thrombotic thrombocytopenic purpura/hemolytic uremic syndrome by protein A immunoadsorption of plasma. Cancer 1993;71:1882–1892.

14. Garibotto G, Acquarone N, Saffioti S, Deferrari G, Villaggio B, Ferrario F. Successful treatment of mitomycin C-associated hemolytic uremic syndrome by plasmapheresis. Nephron 1989;51:409–412.

15. Palmisano J, Agraharkar M, Kaplan AA. Successful treatment of cisplatin induced hemolytic uremic syndrome with thera-

peutic plasma exchange. J Am Soc Nephrol 1997;8:129A. Abstract.

16. Bell WR, Braine HG, Ness PM, Kickler TS. Improved survival of thrombotic thrombocytopenic purpura-hemolytic uremic syndrome: clinical experience in 108 patients. N Engl J Med 1991;325:398–403.

17. Cattran DC. Adult hemolytic-uremic syndrome: successful treatment with plasmapheresis. Am J Kidney Dis 1984;3: 275–279.

18. Agarwal A, Mauer SM, Matas AJ, Nath KA. Recurrent hemolytic uremic syndrome in an adult renal allograft recipient: current concepts and management. J Am Soc Nephrol 1995;6:1160–1169.

HUS in Children

HUS is a major cause of acute renal failure in the pediatric population and often follows an episode of bloody diarrhea as a result of infection with a verotoxin-producing *E. coli* (type 0157-H7) (1,2). The prognosis with supportive therapy is generally good, but a small percentage of patients remains suffering strokes or significant renal failure. A larger number, however, may have evidence for persistent renal involvement as evident by hypertension, proteinuria, and modest decreases in glomerular filtration rate. There have been no randomized controlled trials of plasma exchange as a therapy for childhood HUS; however, controlled trials with plasma infusion have demonstrated only minimal benefit (3). Retrospective analysis and anecdotal reports suggest that plasma exchange may be beneficial in limiting the incidence of significant renal damage in those children considered to be at particularly high risk of irreversible renal damage, such as those who present without a diarrheal prodrome or those older than 5 years of age (4–6). Children with significant central nervous system involvement may also benefit from plasma exchange (7). **Successful TPE prescription for children older than 5 years of age was found to be a median of 4.5 TPE treatments (range, 3 to 10) with a median of 1 liter of plasma exchanged per session (range, 200 to 2000 mL) (4).**

REFERENCES

1. Martin DL, MacDonald KL, White K, Soler JT, Osterholm MT. The epidemiology and clinical aspects of the hemolytic

uremic syndrome in Minnesota. N Engl J Med 1990;323:1161–1167.

2. Rondeau E, Peraldi MN. *Escherichia coli* and the hemolytic uremic syndrome. N Engl J Med 1996;335:660–662. Editorial.
3. Rizzoni G, Claris-Appiani A, Edefonti A, Facchin P, Franchini F, Gusmano R, Imbasciati E, Pavanello L, Perfumo F, Ramuzzi G. Plasma infusion for hemolytic-uremic syndrome in children: results of a multicenter controlled trial. J Pediatr 1988;112: 284–290.
4. Gianviti A, Perna A, Caringella A, Edefonti A, Penza R, Remuzzi G, Rizzoni G. Plasma exchange in children with hemolytic-uremic syndrome at risk of poor outcome. Am J Kidney Dis 1993;22:264–266.
5. Robson WLM, Leung AKC. The successful treatment of atypical hemolytic uremic syndrome with plasmapheresis. Clin Nephrol 1991;35:119–122.
6. Denneberg T, Friedberg M, Holmberg L, Mathiasen C, Nilsson KO, Takolander R, Walder M. Combined plasmapheresis and hemodialysis treatment for severe hemolytic-uremic syndrome following *Campylobacter colitis*. Acta Paediatr Scand 1982;71: 243–245.
7. Sheth KJ, Leichter HE, Gill JC, Baumgardt A. Reversal of central nervous system involvement in hemolytic uremic syndrome by use of plasma exchange. Clin Pediatr 1987;26:651–656.

IDIOPATHIC THROMBOCYTOPENIC PURPURA

ITP results from the presence of antiplatelet antibodies that coat the platelets and lead to their removal by mononuclear phagocytes. Treatment modalities included steroids, splenectomy, immunosuppressive agents, vinca alkaloids, danazol, and intravenous immunoglobulin (IVIG). Several reports describing the use of TPE documented a rapid, but short-lived, increase in platelet counts believed to be related to a concomitant decline in antiplatelet antibodies (1–5). The largest series, a 1-year follow-up of 14 patients, found a lower incidence of relapse in patients treated acutely with TPE and steroids but reported success in only 4 patients because the authors were expecting sustained increases in platelet counts to last for up to 6 months after the termination of treatment (3). It seems that without concomitant therapy, TPE should not be expected to produce sustained remissions, especially with those patients considered to have chronic ITP. In contrast, TPE may be very helpful in producing rapid increases in endogenous platelets and prolonged survival of infused platelets in the immediate presplenectomy period for the purpose of reducing the risk of perioperative hemorrhage. Bussel et al (5) used an imaginative approach combining TPE with IVIG, yielding renewed increases in platelet counts in four of five patients who had become resistant to IVIG alone.

Successful TPE prescriptions have varied, likely reflecting the level of preexisting antiplatelet antibody and, perhaps, the subsequent rapidity of antibody production. **A reasonable initial protocol would involve two to three daily one plasma volume exchanges performed in the immediate preoperative period.** There is at least one report suggesting that **replacement with FFP may yield better results** than replacement with albumin (4), and this approach would seem logical considering the patient's extreme risk of hemorrhage and the anticipated depletion coagulopathy that would result when TPE is replaced with albumin. FFP may also be advantageous because of its content of immunoglobulin, thus mimicking the combined approach promoted by Bussel et al (5).

Refractory ITP has also been reported to respond to "immunomodulation" therapy using a staphylococcal protein A immunoadsorbant system. The Prosorba protein A immunoadsorbant column (Cypress Bioscience, San Diego, CA) is capable of selective adsorption of three subclasses of IgG and may be particularly selective for immune complexes. In contrast to other protein A immunoadsorbant systems (6,7), the Prosorba column is a single-use nonregenerating system and its removal of IgG is relatively modest and reported to be approximately 1 gram per treatment, which must be compared with the 15 to 30 grams of IgG normally removed during a single one plasma volume exchange (8) (see Immunoabsorbant Techniques, Chap. 3). In fact, the relatively minor removal of IgG by the Prosorba column has led to much speculation regarding its presumed mode of action. Possibilities include removal of immune complexes, infusion of anaphylatoxin-producing substances such as activated complement, and stimulation of anti-idiotypic antibodies (9). The Prosorba system is currently approved by the Food and Drug Administration (FDA) for the treatment of idiopathic thrombocytopenic purpura. **Treatment prescription is variable and involves the removal of between 400 and 2000 mL of plasma (separated with any standard TPE device) and perfusion of the plasma over the protein A column** and its subsequent return to the patient. Continuous online plasma separation, plasma perfusion, and subsequent reinfusion can be performed with standard membrane plasma separation, but the process is slow, because the recommended reinfusion rate is only 20 mL/hr. One successful report, describing a favorable response in 5 of 10 ITP patients, describes **weekly treatments** (10). In a larger series, 26 of 72 patients had sustained (greater than 2 months) increases in platelets to more than 50,000/μL (11). Although not statistically significant in the manner analyzed, there appeared to be a greater response in those patients having 2000 mL of plasma treated versus those in whom only 250 mL of plasma was treated. The manufacturer-recommended treatment schedule is one to three procedures per week, for a total of six treatments (12). Usually, minor anaphylactoid reactions (fever, urticarial rash, hypotension) are not uncommon, and a severe treatment-induced vasculitis has been reported (13) such that familiarity with the use and toxicity of this therapy is a prerequisite to its successful application (14). This type of immunoadsorbant therapy may be particularly appealing for the treatment of human immunodeficiency virus–associated thrombocytopenia (15,16).

A recently published clinical guideline from the American Society of Hematology concluded that all available evidence for the use of plasma exchange or plasma infusion must be viewed as being derived from the lowest level of scientific proof (case series with no control group) and should be considered only in severe cases refractory to steroids and splenectomy (17,18).

REFERENCES

1. Branda RF, Tate DY, McCullough JJ, Jacob HS. Plasma exchange in the treatment of fulminant idiopathic (autoimmune) thrombocytopenic purpura. Lancet 1978;1:688–690.
2. Novak R, Wiliams J. Plasmapheresis in catastrophic complications of idiopathic thrombocytopenic purpura. J Pediatr 1978;92:434–435.
3. Marder VJ, Nusbacher J, Anderson FW. One-year follow-up of plasma exchange therapy in 14 patients with idiopathic thrombocytopenic pupura. Transfusion 1981;21:291–297.
4. Porter CC, Ruley EJ, Luban NLC, Phillips TM, Bock GH, Salcedo JR, Fivush BA. Accelerated recovery from immune-mediated thrombocytopenia with plasmapheresis. Am J Med 1985;79:765–768.

5. Bussel JB, Saal S, Gordon B. Combined plasma exchange and intravenous gammaglobulin in the treatment of patients with refractory immune thrombocytopenic purpura. Transfusion 1988;28:38–41.

6. Gjorstrup P, Watt RM. Therapeutic protein A immunoadsorption. A review. Transfus Sci 1990;11:281–302.

7. Samtleben W, Schmidt B, Gurland HJ. Ex vivo and in vivo protein A perfusion: background, basic investigations and first clinical experiences. Blood Purif 1987;5:179–192.

8. Kaplan AA. Towards a rational prescription of plasma exchange: the kinetics of immunoglobulin removal. Semin Dial 1992;5:227–229.

9. Snyder HW Jr, Balint JP, Jones FR. Modulation of immunity in patients with autoimmune disease and cancer treated by extracorporeal immunoadsorption with Prosorba columns. Semin Hematol 1989;26:31–41.

10. Guthrie TH, Oral A. Immune thrombocytopenia purpura: a pilot study of staphylococcal protein A immunomodulation in refractory patients. Semin Hematol 1989;26(suppl 1):3–9.

11. Snyder HW, Cochran SK, Balint JP, Bertram JH, Mittelman A, Guthrie TH, Jones FR. Experience with Prosorba A-immunoadsorption in treatment resistant immune thrombocytopenia. Blood 1992;79:2237–2245.

12. McLeod BC, Strauss RG, Ciavarella D, Gilcher RO, Kasprisin DO, Kiprov DD, Klein HG. Management of hematologic disorders and cancer. J Clin Apheresis 1993;8:211–230.

13. Case records of the Massachusetts General Hospital. N Engl J Med 1994;331:792–800.

14. Snyder HW, Henry DH, Messerschmidt GL, et al. Minimal toxicity during protein A immunoadsorption treatment of malignant disease: an outpatient therapy. J Clin Apheresis 1991; 6:1–10.

15. Snyder H Jr, Bertram JH, Henry DH, Kiprov DD, Benny WB, Mittelman A, Messerschmidt GL, Cochran SK, Perkins W, Balint Jr JP, Jones FR. Use of protein A immunoadsorption as a treatment for thrombocytopenia in HIV-infected homosexual men: a retrospective evaluation of 37 cases. AIDS 1991;5:1257–1260.

16. Mittleman A, Bertram J, Henry DH, Snyder Jr HW, Messerschmidt GL, Ciavarella D, Ainsworth S, Kiprov D, Arlin Z. Treatment of patients with HIV thrombocytopenia and hemolytic uremic syndrome with protein A (Prosorba column)

immunoadsorption. Semin Hematol 1989;26(suppl a):15–18.

17. George JN, Woolf SH, Raskob GE, Wasser JS, Aledort LM, Ballem PJ, et al. Idiopathic thrombocytopenic purpura: a practice guideline developed by explicit methods for the American Society of Hematology. Blood 1996;88:3–40.

18. Diagnosis and treatment of idiopathic thrombocytopenic purpura: recommendations of the American Society of Hematology ITP Practice Guideline Panel. Ann Intern Med 1997;126:319–326.

POST-TRANSFUSION PURPURA

Post-transfusion purpura is a rare cause of immune-mediated thrombocytopenia that is considered to be an anamnestic response to blood transfusion in a previously sensitized patient. The disorder is considered to be the result of the infusion of platelet-associated (PA)-1a antigen-positive platelets in patients with preformed antibody to PA-1a antigen. Severe life-threatening thrombocytopenia can occur approximately 1 week after transfusion. An early report described success with exchange transfusion (1), but TPE is considered less likely to incur antigen-antibody reactions and **successful management has been attained with TPE performed on 3 successive days, each equaling approximately 1.4 to 2 liters** (2). A subsequent report described that a single TPE treatment, approximating 3.3 liters exchanged with FFP, was capable of providing a rapid increase in platelet count in a patient resistant to high-dose corticosteroid therapy (3). A recurrence of thrombocytopenia 10 days after TPE therapy may have been the result of intravascular redistribution of preformed antibody that had been sequestered in the extravascular space, suggesting that a repeat TPE treatment may be required. More recently, this syndrome has been shown to respond rapidly to IVIG therapy (4), which must be considered as a more convenient and more readily available therapy (5). Nonetheless, TPE is still reported as a successful means of treating the disorder (6).

REFERENCES

1. Cimo PL, Aster RH. Post transfusion purpura: successful treatment by exchange transfusion. N Engl J Med 1972;287: 290–292.

2. Abramson N, Eisenberg PD, Aster RH. Post-transfusion purpura: immunologic aspects and therapy. N Engl J Med 1974;291: 1163–1166.

3. Lau P, Sholtis CM, Aster RH. Post-transfusion purpura: an enigma of alloimmunization. Am J Hematol 1980;9:331–336.

4. Mueller-Eckhardt C, Kuenzlen DC, Thilo-Korner D, Pralle H. High dose intravenous immunoglobulin for post-transfusion purpura. N Engl J Med 1983;308:287. Letter.

5. McLeod BC, Strauss RG, Ciavarella D, Gilcher RO, Kasprisin DO, Kiprov DD, Klein HG. Management of hematologic disorders and cancer. J Clin Apheresis 1993;8:211–230.

6. Gonzalez J, Schwartz J, Gerstein G, Klainer AS, Bisaccia E. Case report: post-transfusion purpura. N J Med 1996;93:101–102.

AUTOIMMUNE HEMOLYTIC ANEMIA

Cold Agglutinins

Cold agglutinin–mediated hemolytic anemia may follow certain infections (mycoplasma or immunoblastic lymphadenopathy). TPE has been used to help lower the agglutinin titer and control treatment-resistant hemolysis (1,2). **Successful TPE prescriptions have been modest, usually one or two TPE treatments, of approximately 4 liters of exchange**, to reduce hemolysis of transfused blood. These modest exchange volumes are not inconsistent with the mostly intravascular distribution of the IgM cold agglutinins. It is also **recommended that the apheresis procedure should be performed in a room whose ambient temperature is maintained at 37°C**.

Warm Agglutinins

TPE has also been used successfully in the management of steroid- and splenectomy-resistant idiopathic autoimmune hemolytic anemia, not mediated by cold agglutinins (3–5). In one case, **a single 4.2-liter exchange allowed stabilization of hematocrits for approximately 7 days (3)**. Twenty-eight days later, after initiation of azathioprine, TPE was repeated, with gradual subsidence of hemolysis and ultimate taper of both steroids and azathioprine. In another case, an IgG-mediated hemolytic anemia resistant to steroids, cyclophosphamide, azathioprine, and IVIG responded rapidly to three **TPE treatments exchanging 4000 mL of plasma with albumin (4)**. More recently, there has been a preliminary report of a sustained remission of treatment-resistant hemolytic anemia by the synchronized use of TPE followed by cyclophosphamide (6), similar to scheduling proposed by Schroeder and Euler (7).

A recent review of the available anecdotal reports concluded that normal TPE treatments are most likely to achieve only a short-lived response in warm agglutinin-associated hemolysis and suggested that TPE should be reserved for fulminant cases (8). **Recommended prescription is three to five treatments per week, averaging 1 to 1.5 plasma volumes per exchange.**

REFERENCES

1. Isbister JP, Biggs JC, Penny R. Experience with large volume plasmapheresis in malignant paraproteinemia and immune disorders. Aust N Z J Med 1978;8:154–164.
2. Taft EG, Propp RP, Sullivan SA. Plasma exchange for cold agglutinin hemolytic anemia. Transfusion 1977;17:173–176.
3. Bernstein ML, Schneider BK, Naiman JL. Plasma exchange in refractory acute autoimmune hemolytic anemia. J Pediatr 1981; 98:774–775.
4. Kutti J, Wadenvik H, Safai-Kutti S, Bjorkander J, Hanson LA, Westberg G, Johnsen SA, Larsson B. Successful treatment of refractory autoimmune hemolytic anemia by plasmapheresis. Scand J Haematol 1984;32:149–152.
5. von Keyserlingk H, Meyer-Sabellek W, Arntz R, Haller H. Plasma exchange treatment in autoimmune hemolytic anemia of the warm antibody type with renal failure. Vox Sang 1987;52: 298–300.
6. Silva VA, Ramos RR, Curtis BR, Sadler JE, Chaplin H. Conventional and high dose steroid, splenectomy, intravenous immunoglobulin and pulse cyclophosphamide resistant autoimmune hemolytic anemia successfully treated with plasma exchange followed by pulse and daily oral cyclophosphamide. Presented at the 12th Annual Meeting of the American Society for Apheresis, New Orleans, 1991.
7. Schroeder JO, Euler HH, Loffler H. Synchronization of plasmapheresis and pulse cyclophosphamide in severe systemic lupus erythematosus. Ann Intern Med 1987;107:344–346.
8. McLeod BC, Strauss RG, Ciavarella D, Gilcher RO, Kasprisin DO, Kiprov DD, Klein HG. Management of hematologic disorders and cancer. J Clin Apheresis 1993;8:211–230.

MATERNAL-FETAL INCOMPATIBILITY: Rh DISEASE

Several reports suggested that intensive plasma exchange can successfully lower the level of maternal antibodies directed against fetal blood antigens (1–4). Most of these successful attempts have used **2- to 5-liter weekly exchanges,** but one group, which monitored results with multiple amniocentesis procedures, recommended 10 to 20 liters per week (3). Subsequently, it has been suggested that repeated amniocentesis may have resulted in fetal-maternal blood mixing, causing enhanced immunization and requiring a more aggressive exchange prescription to maintain lowered antibody levels (5). Another potential cause of increased antibody production is contamination of maternal blood with residual amounts of red cells present in the FFP used as the replacement fluid. It is therefore recommended that infused FFP should be from Rh-negative donors. A recent review of the subject concluded that, if used (see below), **TPE should be initiated at a rate of two to three times weekly with 1 to 1.5 plasma volume exchanges (6).** Having listed these recommendations, it should be noted that widespread prevention of Rh immunization and technical advances in umbilical cord sampling and intrauterine transfusion have dramatically reduced the indications for TPE in preventing Rh hemolytic disease. At present, **TPE should be reserved for the situation in which the mother has been immunized against a blood antigen for which the father is homozygous and in which the mother has had a previous history of hydrops at or before 24 to 26 weeks of pregnancy** (7). In this situation, **TPE should begin at 10 to 12 weeks of gestation** when maternal-fetal transfer of IgG is beginning. Amniocentesis or fetal sampling is recommended at 18 to 22 weeks.

REFERENCES

1. Clarke CA, Elson CJ, Bradley J, Donohoe WTA, Lehane D, Hughes-Jones NC. Intensive plasmapheresis as a therapeutic measure in rhesus-immunized women. Lancet 1970;1:793–798.
2. Fraser ID, Bothamley JE, Bennett MO, Airth GR, Lehane D, McCarthy M, Roberts FM. Intensive antenatal plasmapheresis in severe rhesus isoimmunisation. Lancet 1976;1:6–8.
3. Graham-Pole J, Barr W, Willoughby MLN. Continuous-flow plasmapheresis in management of severe rhesus disease. Br Med J 1977;1:1185–1188.

4. Angela E, Robinson E, Tovey LA. Intensive plasma exchange in the management of severe Rh disease. Br J Haematol 1980;45:621–631.
5. Grant CJ, Hamblin TJ, Smith DS, Wellstead L. Plasmapheresis in Rh hemolytic disease: the danger of amniocentesis. Int J Artif Organs 1983;6:83–86.
6. McLeod BC, Strauss RG, Ciavarella D, Gilcher RO, Kasprisin DO, Kiprov DD, Klein HG. Management of hematologic disorders and cancer. J Clin Apheresis 1993;8:211–230.
7. Bowman JM. Hemolytic disease (erythroblastosis fetalis). In: Creasy RK, Resnik R, eds. Maternal-fetal medicine. Philadelphia: WB Saunders, 1994:711–743.

HEMOPHILIA: REMOVAL OF FACTOR VIII INHIBITORS

Factor VIII inhibitors are antibodies that are most commonly found in hemophiliacs but can also occur in women after childbirth and in certain autoimmune diseases. A quantitative assessment of the degree of inhibition can be made in terms of Bethesda units (BU). Patients with titers less than 5 BU may respond to large doses of factor VIII concentrates (100 IU/kg), whereas those with values between 5 and 50 BU may respond only to very large doses (100–150 IU/kg) (1). Plasmapheresis has been reported to be effective for the removal of factor VIII inhibitors, allowing renewed responsiveness to factor VIII infusions (2,3). Appropriate candidates for TPE therapy are those patients resistant to infusion of factor VIII or other hemostatic-inducing concentrates and in whom there is life-threatening hemorrhage or a need for establishing hemostasis in the perioperative period (1,4,5). Effective **TPE prescription has varied from two exchanges in a 3-day period to achieve presurgery hemostasis to 14 daily exchanges for the management of severe postoperative hemorrhage** (2,3). The recommended **exchange volume is 4 liters** *replaced with FFP* to avoid the expected depletion coagulopathy. For maximum effect, the largest dose of factor VIII should be infused immediately after the TPE treatment, followed by smaller doses at 8 or 12 hourly intervals. Most recently, Rubinger et al (6) described the use of TPE as an adjunct therapy during the continuous infusion of porcine factor VIII in patients with factor VIII inhibitors.

Immunoadsorption of factor VIII inhibitor antibodies and induction of immune tolerance to factor VIII infusions have been achieved using a regenerating protein A immunoadsorption column and combined therapy with IVIG and cyclophosphamide (7). Immunoadsorption has the distinct advantage of removing only the antibody and avoiding the expected depletion coagulopathy that necessitates the infusion of FFP. Effective lowering of the antibody titers requires a special device that uses two alternately regenerating columns of protein A (Excorim; Gambro, Lund, Sweden) and would be unlikely with the relatively insignificant IgG removal capabilities of the Prosorba column (see Immunoadsorbant Techniques, Chap. 3). Unfortunately, the Excorim-regenerating immunoadsorption system is not yet FDA approved for use in the United States.

TPE or immunoadsorption may also be useful for the removal of antibody inhibitors directed against other coagulation factors (1).

REFERENCES

1. McLeod BC, Strauss RG, Ciavarella D, Gilcher RO, Kasprisin DO, Kiprov DD, Klein HG. Management of hematologic disorders and cancer. J Clin Apheresis 1993;8:211–230.
2. Slocombe GW, Newland AC, Colvin MP, Colvin BT. The role of intensive plasma exchange in the prevention and management of haemorrhage in patients with inhibitors to factor VIII. Br J Haematol 1981;47:577–585.
3. Bona RD, Pasquale DN, Kalish RI, et al. Porcine factor VIII and plasmapheresis in the management of hemophilia patients with inhibitors. Am J Hematol 1986;21:201–207.
4. American Medical Association Council on Scientific Affairs. Current status of therapeutic plasmapheresis. JAMA 1985;253:819–825.
5. Shumak KH, Rock GA. Therapeutic plasma exchange. N Engl J Med 1984;310:762–771.
6. Rubinger M, Houston DS, Schwetz N, Woloschuk DM, Israels SJ, Johnston JB. Continuous infusion of porcine factor VIII in the management of patients with factor VIII inhibitors. Am J Hematol 1997;56:112–118.
7. Nilsson IM, Berntorp E, Zettervoll O. Induction of immune tolerance in patients with hemophilia and antibodies to factor VIII by combined treatment with intravenous IgG, cyclophosphamide and factor VIII. N Engl J Med 1988;318:947–950.

Metabolic Disorders

9

Hypercholesterolemia   139
  Familial Hypercholesterolemia   140
  Primary Biliary Cirrhosis   141
Hypertriglyceridemia   144
Pruritis Associated with Cholestasis   144
Hepatic Failure   145
Graves' Disease and Thyroid Storm   147
  Graves' Ophthalmopathy   148
Autoantibodies to the Insulin Receptor   149

Proposed indications for therapeutic plasma exchange (TPE) in metabolic disorders are listed in Table 9-1. Because its major morbidity is neurologic, Refsum's disease is listed in the section on neurologic disorders.

HYPERCHOLESTEROLEMIA

Severe hypercholesterolemia resistant to dietary and drug therapy can be seen in familial hypercholesterolemia (type IIa) and primary biliary cirrhosis (PBC). Patients with familial hypercholesterolemia have accelerated atherosclerosis and are prone to early death from myocardial infarction. PBC can result in extremely elevated cholesterol levels, in some cases exceeding 1000 mg/dL. The most common cholesterol-related morbidity in PBC is xanthomatous neuropathy.

Table 9-1. Metabolic Indications for TPE

	Reference and Year		
	1 1986	2 1993	3 1994
		Rating	
Metabolic disorders			
Hypercholesterolemia	II	I–II	I
Hypertriglyceridemia	nl	nl	nl
Pruritis associated with cholestasis	II	nl	nl
Hepatic failure	III	III	nl
Graves' disease and thyroid storm	I	III	III
Insulin receptor antibodies	nl	nl	nl

Rating: I, standard therapy, acceptable but not mandatory; II, available evidence tends to favor efficacy: conventional therapy usually tried first; III, inadequately tested at this time; IV, no demonstrated value in controlled trials. nl, not listed.

REFERENCES: 1. American Medical Association Council on Scientific Affairs. Current status of therapeutic plasmapheresis. JAMA 1985;253:819–825.

2. Strauss RG, Ciavarella D, Gilcher RO, Kasprisin DO, Kiprov DD, Klein HG, McLeod BC. An overview of current management. J Clin Apheresis 1993;8:189–194.

3. Leitman SF, Ciavarella D, McLeod B, Owen H, Price T, Sniecinski I. Guidelines for therapeutic hemapheresis. Bethesda, MD: American Association of Blood Banks, revised 1994.

Familial Hypercholesterolemia

The ability of TPE to reduce the time-averaged cholesterol level in familial hypercholesterolemia is well established (1–4). Most significantly, Thompson et al. (5) reported that five patients undergoing **TPE every other week for a mean of 8.4 years** had a statistically increased mean survival of 5.5 years when compared with their non-TPE-treated homozygous siblings, who presumably had the same genetic defect in low-density-lipoprotein (LDL) receptors. TPE has also been shown to decrease ureteroplacental resistance (decreasing an abnormally high systolic–diastolic ratio) in a pregnant homozygous patient (6). Of note is that during a series of TPE treatments beginning in the fifteenth week of gestation, intratreatment increases in cholesterol were more rapid, necessitating more frequent TPE treatments (from every 4 weeks to every 10 to 14 days).

Although standard plasma exchange can successfully lower serum cholesterol levels, recent interest has been centered on the development of selective lipid removal techniques that can reduce the loss of nonlipid proteins and the desirable high-density lipoproteins that are removed with standard TPE. Three of these systems have undergone extensive clinical trials in the United States (see Selective Plasmapheresis Techniques, Chap. 3). One is an immunoadsorbant system in which plasma is perfused over sepharose beads impregnated with antibodies against LDL (7). Another system uses negatively charged dextran molecules that bind covalently to the positively charged apoprotein B lipoproteins (8). A third method, known as the HELLP system, involves the extracorporeal precipitation of LDL lipoproteins by negatively charged heparin (9). Schaumann et al (10) evaluated all three of these techniques and found them to be similar in biocompatibility and equally efficacious in lowering LDL cholesterol. There are, however, reports of anaphylactoid reactions occurring in patients treated with angiotensin-converting enzyme inhibitors and the dextran sulfate system, suggesting some disorder of bradykinin metabolism (11,12).

An impressive success with these selective lipid removal systems is the report of computer-evaluated coronary angiography that demonstrated atherosclerotic regression in patients treated with drugs and the dextran sulfate system (13). Subsequently, a randomized study comparing simvastatin with and without a biweekly treatment with the dextran sulfate system demonstrated a significant regression in peripheral vascular disease in those treated with the apheresis regimen (14). In agreement with these results, the most recent publications continue to support the concept that aggressive lipid lowering with extracorporeal removal techniques can result in clinically important regression of both coronary and peripheral vascular disease (15–17). One possible "cost-effective" application of this technique would be its short-term use in an attempt to decrease the tendency of postangioplasty patients to reocclude their treated arteries.

Primary Biliary Cirrhosis

In PBC, kinetic analysis has determined that hypercholesterolemia is the result of an excess in synthesis over degradation by as much as 0.4 g/d (18). In comparison, in a patient with a pretreatment value of 415 mg/dL, 6.7 g of cholesterol can be removed with a single one plasma volume exchange (19). Thus, the removal capabilities of repetitive treatments with plasma exchange can exceed production rate and have been documented to result in resolution of xanthomatous collections and remission of neuropathic pain. In 1972, Turnberg et al (18) recommended an initial run of five daily treatments to provide substantial lowering of serum cholesterol levels, which were then maintained with weekly treatment. These treatments were very inefficient, averaging only 500 mL per exchange, and more modern equipment can be effective with a **once weekly schedule exchanging one plasma volume with albumin.** Resolution or improvement in intractable pruritis, common in PBC, is an added benefit provided by TPE (20).

REFERENCES

1. Thompson GR, Lowenthal R, Myant NB. Plasma exchange in management of homozygous familial hypercholesterolemia. Lancet 1975;1:1208–1211.
2. Berger GM, Miller JL, Bonnici F, et al. Continuous flow plasma exchange in the treatment of homozygous familial hypercholesterolemia. Am J Med 1978;65:243–251.
3. King ME, Breslow JL, Lees RS. Plasma exchange therapy of homozygous familial hypercholesterolemia. N Engl J Med 1980;302:1457–1459.
4. Thompson GP. Plasma exchange for hypercholesterolaemia. Lancet 1981;1:1246–1248.
5. Thompson RG, Miller JP, Breslow JL. Improved survival of patients with homozygous familial hypercholesterolaemia treated with plasma exchange. Br Med J 1985;291:1671–1672.
6. Beigel Y, Hod M, Fuchs J, Lurie J, Friedman S, Green P, Merlob P, Melamed R, Ovadia J. Pregnancy in a homozygous familial hypercholesterolemic patient treated with long-term plasma exchange. Am J Obstet Gynecol 1990;162:77–78.
7. Saal SD, Parker TS, Gordon BR. Removal of low-density lipoproteins in patients by extracorporeal immunoadsorption. Am J Med 1986;80:583–589.
8. Gordon BR, Kelsey SF, Bilheimer DW, et al. Treatment of refractory familial hypercholesterolemia by low density lipo-protein apheresis using an automated dextran sulfate cellulose adsorption system. Am J Cardiol 1992;70:1010–1016.
9. Eisenhauer T, Armstrong VW, Schuff-Werner P, et al. Long term clinical experience with HELP-CoA-reductase inhibitors for maximum treatment of coronary heart disease associated with severe hypercholesterolemia. Trans Am Soc Artif Intern Organs 1989;35:580–583.
10. Schaumann D, Olbricht CJ, Welp M, et al. Extracorporeal removal of LDL-cholesterol: prospective evaluation of effec-

tivity, selectivity and biocompatibility. J Am Soc Nephrol 1992;3:392. Abstract.

11. Olbricht CJ, Schaumann D, Fischer D. Anaphylactoid reactions, LDL-pheresis with dextran sulfate and ACE inhibitors. Lancet 1992;340:908–909.

12. Kroon AA, Mol MJTM, Stalenhoff APH. ACE inhibitors and LDL-apheresis with dextran sulfate adsorption. Lancet 1992;340:1476. Letter.

13. Tatami R, Inoue N, Itoh H, Kishino B, Koga N, Nakashima Y, Nishide T, Okamura K, Saito Y, Teramoto T. Regression of coronary atherosclerosis by combined LDL-apheresis and lipid-lowering drug therapy in patients with familial hypercholes-terolemia: a multicenter study. The LAARS Investigators. Atherosclerosis 1992;95:1–13.

14. Kroon AA, van Asten WNJC, Stalenhoef AFH. Effect of apheresis of low-density lipoprotein on peripheral vascular disease in hypercholesterolemic patients with coronary artery disease. Ann Intern Med 1996;125:945–954.

15. Aengevaeren WR, Kroon AA, Stalenhoef AF, Uijen GJ, van der Werf T. Low density lipoprotein apheresis improves regional myocardial perfusion in patients with hypercholesterolemia and extensive coronary artery disease. LDL-Apheresis Atherosclerosis Regression Study (LAARS). J Am Coll Cardiol 1996;28: 1696–1704.

16. Kroon AA, Aengevaeren WR, van der Werf T, Uijen GJ, Reiber JH, Bruschke AV, Stalenhoef AF. LDL-Apheresis Atherosclerosis Regression Study (LAARS). Effect of aggressive versus conventional lipid lowering treatment on coronary atherosclerosis. Circulation 1996;93:1826–1835.

17. Donner MG, Richter WO, Schwandt P. Long term effect of LDL apheresis on coronary heart disease. Eur J Med Res 1997; 2:270–274.

18. Turnberg LA, Mahoney MP, Glesson MH, et al. Plasmaphere-sis and plasma exchange in the treatment of hyperlipidaemia and xanthomatous neuropathy in patients with primary biliary cirrhosis. Gut 1972;13:976–981.

19. Kaplan AA, Halley SE, Reardon J, Sevigny J. One year's expe-rience using a rotating filter for therapeutic plasma exchange. Am Soc Artif Intern Organs Trans 1989;35:262–264.

20. Cohen LB, Ambinder EP, Wolke AM, Field SP, Schaffner F. Role of plasmapheresis in primary biliary cirrhosis. Gut 1985; 26:291–294.

HYPERTRIGLYCERIDEMIA

Familial hypertriglyceridemia may result in triglyceride levels above 1000 mg/dL and an associated risk of acute pancreatitis. In one patient, a mild case of pancreatitis was treated with three one plasma volume exchanges, each resulting in an approximate 60% decline in serum levels. Post-treatment "rebound" was modest, and the combined effect of the three treatments lowered triglyceride levels from 4810 to 238 mg/dL (1). Replacement solution was with 5% albumin. In the same report, the risk of postoperative pancreatitis was reduced by a single TPE treatment that lowered triglyceride levels from 3725 to 587 mg/dL. A more recent report described the successful use of monthly TPE treatments for the prevention of recurrent bouts of pancreatitis in two patients with severe hypertriglyceridemia (types I and V) (2).

Severe hypertriglyceridemia may also be seen in the fat overload syndrome, a rare complication of intravenous fat emulsion administration. It results from an elevation of serum triglyceride levels that can cause microvascular sludging and fat embolization in the lung, brain, kidney, retina, and liver. A severe case with a triglyceride level of 10,000 mg/dL was successfully treated with a single 5.6-liter exchange with FFP (3).

REFERENCES

1. Grima K, Wuest D, Civarella D. Use of therapeutic plasmapheresis in the management of patients with hypertriglyceridemia to prevent or modulate pancreatitis. J Clin Apheresis 1993;8:39. Abstract.
2. Piolot A, Nadler F, Cavallero E, Coquard JL, Jacotot B. Prevention of recurrent acute pancreatitis in patients with severe hypertriglyceridemia: value of regular plasmapheresis. Pancreas 1996; 13:96–99.
3. Kollef MH, McCormack MT, Caras WE, Reddy VVB, Bacon D. The fat overload syndrome: successful treatment with plasma exchange. Ann Intern Med 1990;112:545–546.

PRURITIS ASSOCIATED WITH CHOLESTASIS

Cholestasis-induced pruritis can become an intractable problem in patients with PBC and in those with benign recurrent intrahepatic cholestasis (1). Pathogenesis of the pruritis is unresolved, but retention of bile salts is implicated in most theories. Current treatment options include antihistamines, phenobarbital, cholestyramine, colestipol, naloxone, ursodeoxycholic acid, and ultraviolet light. Pruritis refractory to the above measures may respond to plasma perfusion or standard TPE. Lauterburg et al (1) perfused 1 to 6 liters of plasma over charcoal-coated beads, documenting substantial removal of bile salts and relief from pruritis lasting from 24 hours to 5 months. Cohen et al (2) achieved **prolonged remission by using standard TPE of between 500 and 2000 mL performed three times weekly for 2 weeks and then weekly or biweekly thereafter**. Our own experience suggests that marked relief from pruritis can be achieved with **weekly exchanges involving one plasma volume**. Considering the ever-expanding options for the treatment of cholestasis-induced pruritis, it seems that TPE would be a practical option in only a very few cases. Perhaps more likely is that TPE treatment for PBC-related hypercholesterolemia would have the added benefit of bringing symptomatic relief of the associated pruritis (see Hypercholesterolemia, above).

REFERENCES

1. Lauterburg BH, Taswell HF, Pineda AA, Dickson ER, Burgstaler EA, Carlson GL. Treatment of pruritis of cholestasis by plasma perfusion through USP-charcoal-coated glass beads. Lancet 1980;2:53–55.
2. Cohen LB, Ambinder EP, Wolke AM, Field SP, Schaffner F. Role of plasmapheresis in primary biliary cirrhosis. Gut 1985;26: 291–294.

HEPATIC FAILURE

From a clinical point of view, fulminant hepatic failure leads to two major problems: inability to produce coagulation factors and the failure to detoxify potential neurotoxins. Hence, the two major morbidities of hepatic failure are bleeding and coma. TPE has the potential for the removal of albumin-bound toxins and those that are intrinsically of a large molecular size, such as endotoxin. TPE also allows the massive replacement of blood products for the correction of coagulopathy. Unfortunately, net clearance rates are relatively small, averaging only 3 to 5 liters per treatment, rendering TPE a useful treatment only for those substances with a limited volume of distribution and a relatively slow production rate. Although removed in the discarded plasma during TPE, small- and middle-molecular-weight toxins, which may be involved in the pathophysiology of hepatic failure, are inefficiently removed by TPE because of their relatively large volumes of distribution and their rapid rates of production.

Early reports suggested that TPE could be useful as a means of reversing hepatic coma in patients with fulminant hepatitis (1,2). More extensive experience, however, failed to demonstrate a significant benefit to standard TPE (3). Recently, several Japanese investigators combined TPE and hemofiltration as a means of removing small-, middle-, and large-molecular-weight toxins while at the same time allowing adequate replacement of blood products to control bleeding (4–7). Yoshiba et al (4) reported on the results of 27 patients treated with a combination of **between 2.4 and 4.8 liters of TPE replaced with FFP and between 6 and 30 liters of hemofiltration. Surviving patients received from 3 to 75 treatment sessions (mean, 16 sessions over 19 days).** Ninety-three percent regained consciousness, whereas 55% survived (50% with type A hepatitis, 67% with type B, and 50% with non-A, non-B hepatitis). This aggressive combination approach appears to produce a sufficiently sustained survival to be useful as a bridge to transplant or as a means of supporting those patients in whom there is an expectation of hepatic regeneration. Alternative treatment strategies currently under investigation include combined filter/sorbent systems and filters lined with hepatocytes (8–12). Reference 12 provides a concise review of extracorporeal blood purification techniques for the treatment of hepatic failure.

REFERENCES

1. Lepore MJ, Martel AJ. Plasmapheresis in hepatic coma. Lancet 1967;2:771–772.
2. Lepore MJ, Martel AJ. Plasmapheresis with plasma exchange in hepatic coma. Ann Intern Med 1970;72:165–174.
3. Lepore MJ, Stutman LJ, Bonanno CA, Conklin EF, Robilotti JG, McKenna PJ. Plasmapheresis with plasma exchange in hepatic coma. Arch Intern Med 1972;129:900–907.
4. Yoshiba M, Sekiyama K, Iwamura Y, Sugata F. Development of reliable artificial liver support (ALS)-plasma exchange in combination with hemodiafiltration using high-performance membranes. Dig Dis Sci 1993;38:469–476.

5. Yoshiba M, Sekiyama K, Inoue K. Development of reliable artificial liver support—plasma exchange in combination with hemodiafiltration using high performance membranes. Presented at the Proceedings of the Fifth International Congress of the World Apheresis Association. Houston, March 1994.

6. Matsubara S, Kenji O, Kiyoaki O, Miyazaki Y, Yajima Y, Suzuki H, Otsuki M, Matsuno S. Continuous removal of middle molecules by hemofiltration in patients with acute liver failure. Crit Care Med 1990;18:1331–1338.

7. Matsubara S, Okabe K, Ouchi K, Sato T, Matsuno S. Temporary metabolic support by extracorporeal blood therapy for liver failure after surgery. Am Soc Artif Intern Organs Trans 1988;34:266–269.

8. Stange J, Mitzner S, Straub M, Fischer U, Lindemann S, Peters E, Holtz M, Drewelow B, Schmidt R. Primary or established liver cells for a hybrid liver? Am Soc Artif Intern Organs J 1995;41:M310–M315.

9. Ash SR, Blake De, Carr DJ, Carter C, Howard T, Makowka L. Neurologic improvement of patients with hepatic failure and coma during sorbent suspension dialysis. Trans Am Soc Artif Intern Organs 1991;37:M332–M334.

10. Hughes RD, Williams R. Use of sorbent columns and haemofiltration in fulminant hepatic failure. Blood Purif 1993;11:163–169.

11. Schafer DF. Desperate appliances: a short review of therapies for fulminant hepatic failure. Blood Purif 1993;11:158–162.

12. Kaplan AA, Epstein M. Extracorporeal blood purification in the management of hepatic failure. Semin Nephrol 1997;17:576–682.

GRAVES' DISEASE AND THYROID STORM

Graves' disease is associated with the existence of a thyroid-stimulating immunoglobulin resulting in clinical symptoms of hyperthyroidism. Definitive treatment is ablation of the thyroid gland with surgery or radioactive iodine. Acute symptoms can be managed with iodine, propylthiouracil, or methimazole to block thyroid hormone release and beta blockers to minimize the adrenergic response. Twenty-five percent of the active hormone thyroxine circulates in the intravascular compartment and is 99% bound to serum protein. Its normal serum half-life is 7 days, which is shortened to 4.4 days in thyrotoxicosis. Thyroid "storm" or crisis is characterized by hyperpyrexia, delirium, tachycardia, circulatory embarrassment, diarrhea, vomiting, and severe muscle weakness and may be lethal. Because of the above-mentioned kinetic factors, TPE has been used to treat thyroid storm when conventional methods have failed (1). In one report, three patients resistant to medical therapy responded rapidly to plasma exchange (2). In each case, **2500 to 3500 mL of plasma was exchanged with albumin**. In another report, **one to three TPE treatments were performed to aid in the management of pregnant women with treatment-resistant thyrotoxicosis** (3). The authors remarked that antithyroid drugs and iodides can cross the placenta and may cause fetal goiter and hypothyroidism, whereas prolonged use of beta blockers may result in a small placenta, intrauterine growth retardation, fetal bradycardia, and hypoglycemia. Thus, TPE becomes a rational management strategy when conventional therapy is unsuccessful or requires excessive dosing.

Graves' Ophthalmopathy

TPE has also been advocated as a treatment for the ophthalmopathy of Graves' disease. There is reason to believe that this disorder may be immunoglobulin mediated, and severe progression can clearly occur despite a euthyroid state. One group of investigators reported substantial benefit in ophthalmopathy in four patients with acute deterioration in which surgical decompression was avoided (4,5). Each patient received three or four TPE treatments with 2- to 3-liter exchanges. Three other patients treated by this group were considered to have chronic symptomatology and did not respond. Subsequently, a controlled study compared the results of 24 patients treated with TPE and immunosuppression and 10 patients treated with immunosuppression alone (6). The TPE-treated patients had their medical regimen preceded by four consecutive TPE treatments involving 2000 mL each. Those in the TPE group had an immediate post-TPE decrease in proptosis (maximum of 6 mm), whereas those receiving immunosuppression alone had a less marked improvement (maximum decrease in proptosis of 3 mm). The authors suggested that the more rapid improvement in the TPE group may have been related to decreases in edema and intraocular pressure resulting from the rapid movement of oncotic pressure associated with the apheresis treatments.

In another series, 18 patients were treated with a mean of 4.4 TPE treatments each, and only 2 responded (7). These authors concluded that TPE should be considered only in those patients with deteriorating eye signs in whom conventional therapy failed.

REFERENCES

1. Kasprisin DO, Strauss RG, Ciavarella D, Gilcher RO, Kiprov DD, Klein HG, McLeod BC. Management of metabolic and miscellaneous disorders. J Clin Apheresis 1993;8:231–241.
2. Ashkar FS, Katims RB, Smoak WM, Gilson AJ. Thyroid storm treatment with blood exchange and plasmapheresis. JAMA 1979;214;1275–1279.
3. Derkson RHWM, van de Wiel A, Poortman J, der Kinderen PJ, Kater L. Plasma-exchange in the treatment of severe thyrotoxicosis in pregnancy. Eur J Obstet Gynecol Reprod Biol 1984; 18:139–148.
4. Dandona P, Marshall NJ, Bidey SP, Nathan AW, Harvard CW. Successful treatment of exophthalmos and pretibia myxedema with plasmapheresis. Br Med J 1979;1:374–376.
5. Dandona P, Marshall NJ, Bidey SP, Nathan AW, Harvard CW. Exophthalmos and pretibial myxedema not responding to plasmapheresis. Br Med J 1979;2:667–668.
6. De Rosa G, Menichella G, Della S, Rossi PL. Testa A, Pierelli L, Cecchini L, Calla C, Mango G. Plasma exchange in Graves' ophthalmopathy. In: Rock G, ed. Apheresis. New York: Wiley-Liss, 1990:321–325.
7. Kelly W, Langson D, Smithhard D, Fawcitt R, Wensley R, Noble J, Keeley J. An evaluation of plasma exchange for Graves' ophthalmopathy. Clin Endocrinol 1983;18:485–493.

AUTOANTIBODIES TO THE INSULIN RECEPTOR

Autoantibodies to the insulin receptor, causing insulin requirements of 10,000 U/day, were successfully removed with 10 TPE treatments performed over a 21-day period (1). Results were measurable after each treatment, but post-treatment antibody rebound was apparent and may have been partially related to a release in tissue-bound antibody. Concomitant therapy with immunosuppressive medications was recommended to limit renewed antibody synthesis.

REFERENCE

1. Muggeo M, Flier JS, Abrams RA, Harrison LC, Deisserroth AB, Kahn CR. Treatment by plasma exchange of a patient with autoantibodies to the insulin receptor. N Engl J Med 1979; 300:477–480.

Dermatologic Disorders

10

Pemphigus Vulgaris   151
Bullous Pemphigoid   154
Toxic Epidermal Necrolysis (Lyell's Syndrome)   155
Porphyria Cutanea Tarda   156
Psoriasis   157

Dermatologic indications for therapeutic plasma exchange (TPE) are listed in Table 10-1. Purpuric disorders associated with thrombocytopenia or cryoglobulinemia are listed in Chapter 8, whereas those skin disorders associated with vasculitides (leukocytoclastic vasculitis) are listed in Chapters 11 and 12 (Henoch-Schönlein purpura is listed in Chap. 12 and rheumatoid vasculitis and other systemic vasculitides are listed in Chap. 11). Because of its great propensity to cause systemic manifestations, scleroderma is listed in Chapter 11.

PEMPHIGUS VULGARIS

Pemphigus vulgaris is a rare and sometimes fatal disease characterized by the appearance of relapsing crops of bullae of the skin and mucous membranes, leading to erosions and ulcerations. Presentation is usually with painful erosions initially in the oral mucosa and progressing to the scalp, face, and trunk. A distinguishing feature is the superficial detachment of normally appearing skin after pressure (Nikolsky's sign). Skin biopsy reveals acantholysis deep in the epidermis, immediately above the basal layer. Immunofluorescence studies are confirmatory and reveal antibodies to intracellular gly-

Table 10-1. Dermatologic Indications for TPE

	Reference and Year		
	1 1986	2 1993	3 1994
		Rating	
Dermatologic disorders			
Pemphigus vulgaris	III	II	nl
Bullous pemphigus	nl	II	nl
Toxic epidermal necrolysis (Lyell's syndrome)	nl	nl	nl
Porphyria cutanea tarda	nl	nl	nl
Psoriasis	III	IV	IV

Rating: I, standard therapy, acceptable but not mandatory; II, available evidence tends to favor efficacy: conventional therapy usually tried first; III, inadequately tested at this time; IV, no demonstrated value in controlled trials. nl, not listed.
REFERENCES: 1. American Medical Association Council on Scientific Affairs. Current status of therapeutic plasmapheresis. JAMA 1985;253:819–825.
2. Strauss RG, Ciavarella D, Gilcher RO, Kasprisin DO, Kiprov DD, Klein HG, McLeod BC. An overview of current management. J Clin Apheresis 1993;8:189–194.
3. Leitman SF, Ciavarella D, McLeod B, Owen H, Price T, Sniecinski I. Guidelines for therapeutic hemapheresis. Bethesda, MD: American Association of Blood Banks, revised 1994.

coprotein antigens. Passive transfer of the disease has been demonstrated after inoculation of mice with patient-derived IgG, strongly implicating a pathogenetic role of the autoantibodies. Medical management includes steroids and immunosuppressive agents (1).

An early uncontrolled study reported that TPE might be useful as an adjunctive therapy in corticoresistant pemphigus (2), but the same group published a subsequent controlled trial of 40 patients in which a benefit from TPE could not be confirmed (3). Unfortunately, on randomization, the TPE-treated group in the controlled trial included 5 of 22 patients in whom there was no detectable serum level of pemphigus antibody, whereas only 1 of 18 patients in the non-TPE group were antibody negative. Furthermore, the controlled trial used corticosteroids exclusively, without use of immunosuppressive agents, which are often considered most useful in controlling antibody production (4). Thus, the potential value for TPE in the management of pemphigus remains unconfirmed by controlled trial, but several investigators reported good results and continue to recommend TPE in the management of patients resistant to more conventional therapy (5,6). Consistent with this approach, a comparative study involving 22 patients demonstrated that patients with detectable serum levels of pemphigus antibody have a more rapid decrease in these levels when TPE is added to steroid and immunosuppressive therapy (7). TPE has also been found useful during pregnancy when cytotoxic drugs are undesirable (8,9). In a recent extensive review, Bystryn and Steinman (10) underscored the concept that the most successful use of TPE is when it is coupled with immunosuppressive therapy, such as cyclophosphamide. In an assessment of all available treatment options, they concluded that TPE appears to be worthwhile in patients with severe pemphigus unresponsive to conventional therapy.

TPE may be most useful during acute stages of the disease or to help lower the dose of maintenance steroids or cytotoxic drugs. **Recommended prescription during exacerbations is three to five daily TPE treatments in a 1-week period, exchanging 1 to 1.5 plasma volumes (5,6,11).** Patients with severe or refractory disease may require more than five treatments. Replacement fluid can be with albumin.

REFERENCES

1. Fine JD. Management of acquired bullous skin diseases. N Engl J Med 1995;333:1475–1484.
2. Roujeau JC, Andre C, Fabre MJ, Lauret P, Flechet ML, Kalis B, Revuz J, Touraine R. Plasma exchange in pemphigus: an uncontrolled study. Arch Dermatol 1983;119:215–221.
3. Guillaume JC, Roujeau JC, Morel P, Soutre MS, Guillot B, Lambert D, Lauret P, Lorette G, Prigent F, Triller R, Vaillant L. Controlled study of plasma exchange in pemphigus. Arch Dermatol 1988;124:1659–1663.
4. Euler HH, Loffler H, Christophers E. Synchronization of plasmapheresis and pulse cyclophosphamide therapy in pemphigus vulgaris. Arch Dermatol 1987;123:1205–1210.
5. Bystryn JC. Plasmapheresis therapy of pemphigus. Arch Dermatol 1988;124:1702–1704.
6. Roujeau JC, Kalis B, Lauret P, Flechet ML, Fabre MJ, Andre C, Revuz J, Touraines R. Plasma exchange in corticosteroid-resistant pemphigus. Br J Dermatol 1982;106:103–104.
7. Tan-Lim R, Bystryn JC. Effect of plasmapheresis therapy on circulating levels of pemphigus antibodies. J Am Acad Dermatol 1990;22:35–40.

8. Metzker A, Merlob P. Pemphigus in pregnancy: a reevaluation of fetal risk. Am J Obstet Gynecol 1987;157:1012–1013. Letter.
9. Metzker A, Merlob P. Pemphigus in pregnancy. Am J Obstet Gynecol 1990;163:1097. Letter; Comments.
10. Bystryn JC, Steinman NM. The adjuvant therapy of pemphigus. An update. Arch Dermatol 1996;132:203–212.
11. Kiprov DD, Strauss RG, Ciavarella D, Gilcher RO, Kasprisin DO, Klein HG, McLeod BC. Management of autoimmune disorders. J Clin Apheresis 1993;8:195–210.

BULLOUS PEMPHIGOID

Bullous pemphigoid is an autoimmune disease associated with chronic blistering skin lesions occurring primarily in older patients. Histologically, it is associated with linear deposition of IgG and complement in the basement membrane zone of the dermoepidermal junction. As opposed to the more serious pemphigus vulgaris, however, there is no acantholysis. Treatment is usually with steroids, but TPE has been a useful adjunct to therapy in certain resistant cases (1). In a randomized study involving 41 patients treated with steroids alone or with the addition of TPE, 13 of 22 patients treated with TPE were able to achieve disease control with a substantially reduced dose of steroids (2). TPE was prescribed as **eight exchanges over a 4-week period, each involving 60 mL/kg**. Other anecdotal reports suggested that TPE may be helpful in achieving remissions in severe disease (3,4). In one of these, laryngeal involvement leading to respiratory arrest was apparently resistant to both methylprednisolone and azathioprine but responded favorably to three TPE treatments exchanging 3000 mL each (4).

REFERENCES

1. Fine JD. Management of acquired bullous skin diseases. N Engl J Med 1995;333:1475–1484.
2. Roujeau J-C, Guillaume J-C, Morel P, Crickx B, Dalle D, Doutre M-S, Guillot B, Godard W, Gorin I, Labeille B, Lorette G, Rifle G, Souteyrand P, Triller R, Revuz J. Plasma exchange in bullous pemphigoid. Lancet 1984;2:486–489.
3. Goldberg NS, Robinson JK, Roenigk HH Jr, Marder R, Rothe M. Plasmapheresis therapy for bullous pemphigoid. Arch Dermatol 1985;121:1484–1485.

4. Konstadt JW, Remlinger K, Schild J, Aronson I, Bennin B, Solomon L. Refractory bullous pemphigoid leading to respiratory arrest and successfully treated with plasmapheresis. Arch Dermatol 1990;126:1241–1242.

TOXIC EPIDERMAL NECROLYSIS (LYELL'S SYNDROME)

Drug-induced toxic epidermal necrolysis (TEN) is a fulminant potentially lethal disease in which there is widespread epithelial necrosis of skin and mucous membranes. Bullae and erosions can involve between 20 and 100% of the total body surface area. Commonly implicated drugs include barbiturates, phenytoin, sulfonamides, and nonsteroidal anti-inflammatory agents. Medical management includes large volumes of fluids and electrolytes to replace skin losses and aggressive topical skin care (1). Kamanabroo et al (2) reported on the use of TPE as an adjunctive treatment for TEN in five patients. The authors claimed dramatic improvement after **one to three TPE treatments**. In theory, TPE could remove the inciting drug, its metabolites, or some "necrolytic factor." Despite the encouraging results, a review of the data concluded that the role of TPE could not be determined, because the study involved too few patients, was uncontrolled, and had insufficient information regarding the degree of cutaneous involvement (3).

Subsequently, two further reports suggested a positive effect of TPE. Sakellariou et al (4) described their experience with five patients, three of whom had involvement of almost the entire body surface. The mouth, esophagus, and lungs were also involved. Suspected etiologic agents included carbamazepine, paracetamol, a combination of paracetamol and mefenamic acid, allopurinol, and ciprofloxacin. Steroids proved ineffective, prompting the use of TPE. One to five treatments were performed. Complete remission of the syndrome was achieved in four patients, whereas the remaining patient died from septic shock. Most recently, Chaidemenos et al (5) reported on their experience with seven patients presenting with TEN involving 30 to 80% of body surface area and two or four mucous membranes. Suspected etiologic factors were malignancy (Hodgkin's disease and brain tumor) and drugs (carbamazepine, allopurinol, diphenylhydantoin, cefaclor, and amoxicillin with clavullanic acid). **One to four TPE treatments involving 2.5 liters each were performed on alternate days in six patients and on a daily basis in the seventh.** All patients recovered with no new lesions appearing after the first TPE in four patients. There were no adverse reactions to the TPE treatments. After a follow-up period of up to 8 years, no sequelae were noted from the TEN. The authors concluded that TPE is expensive but safe and efficacious by providing rapid relief from pain and rapid cessation of necrolysis. They suggested that TPE should be considered as a first-line therapy in TEN.

REFERENCES

1. Fine JD. Management of acquired bullous skin diseases. N Engl J Med 1995;333:1475–1484.
2. Kamanabroo D, Schmitz-Landgraf W, Czarnetzki BM. Plasmapheresis in severe drug-induced toxic epidermal necrolysis. Arch Dermatol 1985;121:1548–1549.
3. Avakian R, Flowers FP, Araujo OE, Ramos-Caro FA. Toxic epidermal necrolysis: a review. J Am Acad Dermatol 1991;25:69–79.
4. Sakellariou G, Koukoudis P, Karpouzas J, Alexopoulos E, Papadopoulou D, Chrisomalis F, Skenteris N, Tsakaris D, Papadimitriou M. Plasma exchange (PE) treatment in drug-induced toxic epidermal necrolysis (TEN). Int J Artif Organs 1991;14:634–638.
5. Chaidemenos GC, Chrysomallis F, Sombolos K, Mourellou O, Ioannides D, Papakonstantinou M. Plasmapheresis in toxic epidermal necrolysis. Int J Dermatol 1997;36:218–221.

PORPHYRIA CUTANEA TARDA

Porphyria cutanea tarda (PCT) results from a decrease in uroporphyrinogen decarboxylase, leading to increased levels of porphyrins in plasma and their deposition in skin, causing vesicles or bullae in sun-exposed areas. An iron-dependent oxidative mechanism inactivates the decarboxylase, and iron removal through phlebotomy is commonly recommended to activate new enzyme synthesis. Phlebotomy in hemodialysis patients may be problematic because of disordered iron metabolism and anemia. Although uroporphyrin is of a relatively low molecular weight, it is protein bound and inefficiently dialyzable; thus, TPE has been proposed as a means of its extraction. Disler et al (1) successfully managed a case of hemodialysis-associated PCT with TPE. **Two TPE treatments were performed 48 hours apart, each treatment involving 4 liters replaced with fresh frozen plasma.** There was a rapid reduction in uroporphyrin after the two treatments from 44.25 to 14.84 μg/dL after the first treatment and to 8.41 μg/dL after the second treatment (normal values, <0.2 μg/dL), but there was a rapid rebound within days to 38.25 μg/dL. Despite the rebound, there was a rapid resolution of the bullous skin lesions with no recurrence after 4 months of follow-up. In contrast to this successful application, Anderson et al (2) found no improvement with TPE and were successful in mobilizing iron stores with erythropoietin and small-volume phlebotomies. Miyauchi et al (3) treated one case of alcohol-related PCT with abstention from alcohol and repeated 250-mL exchanges of plasma with saline. Because phlebotomy is effective, it must be considered the treatment of choice for most cases (4).

REFERENCES

1. Disler P, Day R, Burman N, Blekkenhorst G, Eales L. Treatment of hemodialysis-related porphyria cutanea tarda with plasma exchange. Am J Med 1982;72:989–993.
2. Anderson KE, Goeger DE, Carson RW, Lee SK, Stead RB. Erythropoietin for the treatment of porphyria cutanea tarda in a patient on long-term hemodialysis. N Engl J Med 1990;322: 315–317.
3. Miyauchi S, Shiraishi S, Miki Y. Small volume plasmapheresis in the management of porphyria cutanea tarda. Arch Dermatol 1983;119:752–755.
4. Kasprisin DO, Strauss RG, Ciavarella D, Gilcher RO, Kiprov DD, Klein HG, McLeod BC. Management of metabolic and miscellaneous disorders. J Clin Apheresis 1993;8:231–241.

PSORIASIS

Psoriasis is a common dermatologic disease manifested by erythematous papules covered by silvery scales. In a small number of patients, there may be an associated disabling arthritis. An autoimmune basis for the disease is debated and may be most likely associated with the arthropathy. Several anecdotal reports suggested that TPE is beneficial in severe psoriasis (1), but a controlled trial of mild disease, using weekly 3-liter exchanges, found no benefit (2). Conceptually, if immune complexes play a role in the arthritis, TPE may be beneficial, but several exchanges per week would be required for an adequate decrease in immune complex levels. A recent review of the available literature concluded that TPE must be considered as an unproven experimental treatment (3).

REFERENCES

1. Dau PD. Resolution of psoriasis during plasmapheresis therapy. Arch Dermatol 1979;115:1171.
2. Clemmensen OJ, Andresen R, Andersen E. Plasmapheresis in the treatment of psoriasis. A controlled clinical study. J Am Acad Dermatol 1983;8:190–192.
3. Kasprisin DO, Strauss RG, Ciavarella D, Gilcher RO, Kiprov DD, Klein HG, McLeod BC. Management of metabolic and miscellaneous disorders. J Clin Apheresis 1993;8:231–241.

Rheumatologic Disorders

11

Systemic Lupus Erythematosus   159
Lupus Anticoagulant, Anticardiolipin Antibodies, and the Antiphospholipid Antibody
   Syndrome   163
   Recurrent Fetal Loss   163
   Catastrophic Antiphospholipid Syndrome   164
   Renal Disease   164
Scleroderma   166
Rheumatoid Arthritis and Rheumatoid Vasculitis   169
   Rheumatoid Vasculitis   170
Vasculitis   172
Polymyositis and Dermatomyositis   175
Raynaud's Disease   176

Rheumatologic indications for therapeutic plasma exchange (TPE) are listed and graded in Table 11-1. Because of its potential for renal involvement, Henoch-Schönlein purpura is reviewed in Chapter 12. Cryoglobulinemia is reviewed in Chapter 8.

SYSTEMIC LUPUS ERYTHEMATOSUS

Despite a plethora of early enthusiastic reports suggesting a positive effect of plasma exchange on severe lupus (1–5), several randomized controlled trials could not document any therapeutic benefit of TPE (6–8). The largest and most recent of these involved the randomization of 86 patients with severe lupus nephritis (8). All 86 received similar conventional therapy with prednisone and cyclophosphamide, whereas 40 underwent plasma exchange three times weekly for the first 4 weeks of treatment. Despite a more rapid decline in double-stranded DNA titers, 25% in the TPE-

Table 11-1. Rheumatologic Indications for TPE

| | Reference and Year | | |
	1 1986	2 1993	3 1994
		Rating	
Rheumatologic disorders			
Systemic lupus erythematosus	II	II	nl
Antiphospholipid antibody syndrome (lupus anticoagulant)	nl	nl	nl
Scleroderma	III	III	III
Rheumatoid arthritis and rheumatoid vasculitis	II	III	IV and II
Vasculitis	II	II	II
Polymyositis/dermatomyositis	III	III/IV	IV
Raynaud's disease	III	II	nl

Rating: I, standard therapy, acceptable but not mandatory; II, available evidence tends to favor efficacy: conventional therapy usually tried first; III, inadequately tested at this time; IV, no demonstrated value in controlled trials. nl, not listed.

REFERENCES: 1. American Medical Association Council on Scientific Affairs. Current status of therapeutic plasmapheresis. JAMA 1985;253:819–825.
2. Strauss RG, Ciavarella D, Gilcher RO, Kasprisin DO, Kiprov DD, Klein HG, McLeod BC. An overview of current management. J Clin Apheresis 1993;8:189–194.
3. Leitman SF, Ciavarella D, McLeod B, Owen H, Price T, Sniecinski I. Guidelines for therapeutic hemapheresis. Bethesda, MD: American Association of Blood Banks, revised 1994.

treated group developed renal failure compared with only 17% of those not receiving TPE. Thus, the weight of the currently available evidence suggests that standard regimens of TPE are not beneficial as a general adjunct to conventional immunosuppressive therapy for lupus nephritis. Nonetheless, TPE may still be useful for the treatment of lupus-associated thrombotic thrombocytopenic purpura (9), for the treatment of symptoms associated with the lupus anticoagulant (see below), or as a means of controlling the disease during pregnancy when cytotoxic agents are undesirable (10). A recent review concluded that TPE may still be used in severe resistant cases of lupus-related morbidities, such as vasculitis with central nervous system (CNS) involvement, peripheral neuropathy, hemolytic anemia, idiopathic thrombocytopenic purpura, pneumonitis, and rapidly progressive renal disease (11). In these situations, these reviewers suggested an aggressive approach with **daily** exchanges of 1 to 1.5 plasma volumes to be continued until there is evidence for clinical improvement or laboratory signs of the effect of concomitantly given immunosuppressive agents. If no improvement is noted after 10 daily exchanges, further treatments are unlikely to be successful. It is also recommended that TPE treatments should be tapered gradually over a 4-week period.

There has even been the suggestion that TPE may be detrimental by incurring a rebound antibody production, but the four cases reported were receiving no concomitant therapy (neither steroids nor immunosuppressives) and the described deterioration occurred up to 6 months after the last TPE treatment (12). Indeed, an ongoing international trial has been designed to take advantage of this proposed apheresis-induced antibody rebound with a synchronization of treatment that involves the withdrawal of cytotoxic and steroid therapy, the initiation of 3 days of TPE (60 mL/kg, replaced with albumin), and the subsequent administration of 3 days of pulse cyclophosphamide followed by up to 6 months of oral dosing (13). The basic rationale of the trial is that pathogenic lymphocytes will be stimulated during the postpheresis period, thus being more susceptible to subsequent cyclophosphamide therapy (14). Thus far, over 170 patients have been enrolled from 35 centers in Europe, Canada, and the United States (15). Partial reporting from the study center in Germany has described a rapid beneficial response in all 14 patients undergoing the synchronized protocol, with 8 remaining off all therapy for a mean of 5.6 years (16). Unfortunately, 4 of 14 patients developed irreversible amenorrhea and 1 patient developed a squamous cell carcinoma of the oropharynx within 17 months of treatment initiation. Definitive results of the entire trial have yet to be published, but an interim report is available (17).

REFERENCES

1. Jones JV, Cumming RH, Bucknall RC, Asplin CM, Fraser ID, Bothamley J, Davis P, Hamblin TJ. Plasmapheresis in the management of acute systemic lupus erythematosus? Lancet 1976;1:709–711.
2. Jones JV, Cumming RH, Bacon PA, Evers J, Fraser ID, Bothamley J, Tribe CR, Davis P, Huges GRV. Evidence for a therapeutic effect of plasmapheresis in patients with systemic lupus erythematosus. Q J Med 1979;192:555–576.

3. Jones JV, Robinson MF, Parciany RK, Layfer LF, McLeod B. Therapeutic plasmapheresis in systemic lupus erythematosus. Arthritis Rheum 1981;24:1113–1120.

4. Abdou NI, Lindsley HB, Pollock A, Stechschulte DJ, Wood G. Plasmapheresis in active lupus erythematosus: effect on clinical, serum and cellular abnormalities. Case report. Clin Immunol Immunopath 1981;19:44–54.

5. Leaker BR, Becker GJ, Dowling JP, Kincaid-Smith PS. Rapid improvement in severe lupus glomerular lesions following intensive plasma exchange associated with immunosuppression. Clin Nephrol 1986;25:236–244.

6. Wei N, Klippel JH, Huston DP, Hall RP, Lawley TJ, Balow JE, Steinberg AD, Decker JL. Randomized trial of plasma exchange in mild systemic lupus erythematosus. Lancet 1983;1:17–21.

7. French Collaborative Group. A randomized trial of plasma exchange in severe acute systemic lupus erythematosus: methodology and interim analysis. Transfus Technol 1985; 6:535–539.

8. Lewis EJ, Hunsicker LG, Lan SP, Rohde RD, Lachin JM, and the Lupus Nephritis Collaborative Study Group. A controlled trial of plasmapheresis therapy in severe lupus nephritis. N Engl J Med 1992;326:1373–1379.

9. Stricker R, Davis JA, Gershow J, Yamamoto KS, Kiprov DD. Thrombotic thrombocytopenic purpura complicating systemic lupus erythematosus. Case report and literature review from the plasmapheresis era. J Rheumatol 1992;19:1469–1473.

10. Thomson BJ, Watson ML, Liston WA, Lambie AT. Plasmapheresis in a pregnancy complicated by acute systemic lupus erythematosus. Case report. Br J Obstet 1985;92:532–534.

11. Kiprov DD, Strauss RG, Ciavarella D, Gilcher RO, Kasprisin DO, Klein HG, McLeod BC. Management of autoimmune disorders. J Clin Apheresis 1993;8:195–210.

12. Schlansky R, DeHoratius RJ, Pincus T, Tung KSK. Plasmapheresis in systemic lupus erythematosus: a cautionary note. Arth Rheumatol 1981;24:49–53.

13. Euler HH, Schroeder JO, Zeuner RA, Teske E. A randomized trial of plasmapheresis and subsequent pulse cyclophosphamide in severe lupus: design of the LPSG trial. Int J Artif Organs 1991;14:639–646.

14. Schroeder JO, Euler HH, Loffler H. Synchronization of plasmapheresis and pulse cyclophosphamide in severe systemic lupus erythematosus. Ann Intern Med 1987;107:344–346.

15. LPSG-Lupus Plasmapheresis Study Group. Circular #1. University of Kiel, Kiel, Germany: Clinical Coordinating Center, 1995.
16. Euler HH, Schroeder JO, Harten P, Zeuner RA, Gutschmidt HJ. Treatment-free remission in severe systemic lupus erythematosus following synchronization of plasmapheresis with subsequent pulse cyclophosphamide. Arthritis Rheum 1994; 37:1784–1794.
17. Euler HH, Schwab UM, Schroeder JO, Hasford J. The Lupus Plasmapheresis Study Group: rationale and updated interim report. Artif Organs 1996;20:356–359.

LUPUS ANTICOAGULANT, ANTICARDIOLIPIN ANTIBODIES, AND THE ANTIPHOSPHOLIPID ANTIBODY SYNDROME

The lupus anticoagulant and the anticardiolipin antibody are antiphospholipid antibodies that are associated with the development of recurrent arterial and venous thromboses, thrombocytopenia, recurrent fetal loss, and, on occasion, renal disease. Systemic coagulation can result in multiple organ involvement and the "catastrophic antiphospholipid syndrome" (CAPS). An analysis of 29 published series comprising over 1000 patients with systemic lupus erythematosus (SLE) found a 34% frequency for the lupus anticoagulant and a 44% frequency for the anticardiolipin antibody (1). Nonetheless, 65% of patients with antiphospholipid antibodies do not have lupus or a lupus-like disease. In this group, the most common associations are with other autoimmune diseases, certain drugs (chlorpromazine, procainamide, hydralazine), and neoplastic disorders. Considering that the lupus anticoagulants are IgG, IgA, or IgM antibodies that bind to protein-phospholipid complexes and, by cross-reactivity, to cardiolipin, it is not surprising that several investigators have used TPE as a means of treating the disorder.

Recurrent Fetal Loss

Two reports describe the use of TPE for the removal of antiphospholipid antibodies to avoid spontaneous abortion. Frampton et al (2) performed repeated exchanges approximating **three to four treatments per week starting from the fourteenth week of pregnancy until successful delivery after 34 weeks**, whereas Fulcher et al (3) performed **six exchanges beginning at the twenty-fourth week** followed by successful cesarean section on week 29. In both reports, there was a substantial lowering of the offending antibody after apheresis.

Catastrophic Antiphospholipid Syndrome

Asherson and Piette (4) reported on 31 patients with CAPS as defined as the presence of antiphospholipid antibodies and multiorgan failure. Thirteen suffered from a "primary" antiphospholipid syndrome, 13 from SLE, 4 from "lupus-like" diseases, and 1 from rheumatoid arthritis. Precipitating factors were evident in one-third of the patients (i.e., infections, major/minor surgical procedures, oral contraceptives). Mortality was 60%, resulting from myocardial failure, acute respiratory distress syndrome, or CNS causes. Disseminated intravascular coagulation was present in 8 of 31 patients. Plasmapheresis appeared to be useful in several who had not responded to conventional therapy with intravenous heparin, steroids, and immunosuppression.

Most recently, Neuwelt et al (5) reported on the course of a patient with a past medical history of the HELLP syndrome (hemolysis, elevated liver enzymes, and low platelets; see HELLP Syndrome, Chap. 8) who developed CAPS. Anticoagulants, corticosteroids, intravenous gammaglobulin, and cyclophosphamide had all failed to halt the progression of CAPS, but over a 3-year period, repeated plasmapheresis treatment halted the condition and led to a reversal of an associated leukoencephalopathy.

Renal Disease

Although most patients with SLE–associated nephritis and antiphospholipid antibodies will have renal disease compatible with the standard World Health Organization classification of lupus nephritis (6–8), there will be a subset whose glomerular pathology is associated with intraglomerular thrombi characteristic of a thrombotic microangiopathy. In an indepth study of the different types of antiphospholipid antibodies and lupus nephritis, Frampton et al (6) found no major pathogenetic role for the antiphospholipid antibodies but did find an association between IgG antiphospholipid antibodies and the presence of intraglomerular thrombi. Reports of the use of TPE for removal of antiphospholipid antibodies in renal disease are scarce. Farrugia et al (8) reported that one of their patients with lupus anticoagulant and renal disease was treated with plasmapheresis, and Kincaid-Smith et al (9) described 12 patients with lupus anticoagulant–associated thrombotic microangiopathy related to pregnancy in which complete renal recovery was only obtained in the two patients treated with TPE. Unfortunately, neither of these reports described the apheresis prescription or the resulting changes in anticoagulant levels.

Despite the paucity of details regarding the use of TPE for renal disease, if antiphospholipid antibodies are associated with an intraglomerular thrombotic microangiopathy, the available data do suggest the possibility of improving renal outcome with the successful lowering of the antiphospholipid antibody levels. Indeed, our own experience demonstrated success in reducing or eliminating the previously elevated levels of these antibodies. Actual prescription of TPE will depend on the individual patient presentation, but **a reasonable schedule is three to five treatments over a 7-day period**. It should be noted that monitoring for the presence of the lupus anticoagulant using the simple prolongation of the partial thromboplastin time (PTT) (10) will be invalid once apheresis is initiated because of the expected "depletion coagulopathy," resulting in a marked prolongation of the PTT. Under these conditions, the presence of the antiphospholipid antibody must be determined by specific antibody testing (11). Concomitant treatment with anticoagulants, steroids, or immunosuppressive agents should be considered in each individual case.

REFERENCES

1. Love PE, Santoro SA. Antiphospholipid antibodies: anticardiolipin and the lupus anticoagulant in systemic lupus erythematosus (SLE) and in non-SLE disorders. Prevalence and clinical significance. Ann Intern Med 1990;112:682–698.
2. Frampton G, Cameron JS, Thom M, Jones S, Raftery M. Successful removal of antiphospholipid antibody during pregnancy using plasma exchange and low dose prednisolone. Lancet 1987;2:1023–1024.
3. Fulcher D, Stewart G, Exner T, Trudinger B, Jeremy R. Plasma exchange and the anticardiolipin syndrome in pregnancy. Lancet 1989;2:171.
4. Asherson RA, Piette JC. The catastrophic antiphospholipid syndrome 1996: acute multi-organ failure associated with antiphospholipid antibodies: a review of 31 patients. Lupus 1996;5:414–417.
5. Neuwelt CM, Daikh DI, Linfoot JA, Pfister DA, Young RG, Webb RL, London SS, Asherson RA. Catastrophic antiphos-

pholipid syndrome: response to repeated plasmapheresis over three years. Arthritis Rheum 1997;40:1534–1539.

6. Frampton G, Hicks J, Cameron JS. Significance of anti-phospholipid antibodies in patients with lupus nephritis. Kidney Int 1991;39:1225–1231.

7. Kincaid-Smith P, Nicholls K. Renal thrombotic microvascular disease associated with LAC. Nephron 1990;54:285–288.

8. Farrugia E, Torres VE, Gastineau D, Michet CJ, Holley KE. Lupus anticoagulant in SLE: a clinical and renal pathological study. Am J Kidney Dis 1992;20:463–471.

9. Kincaid-Smith P, Fairley K, Kloss M. Lupus anticoagulant associated with renal thrombotic microangiopathy and pregnancy related renal failure. Q J Med 1988;258:795–815.

10. Glueck HI, Kant KS, Weiss MA, Pollak VE, Miller MA, Coots M. Thrombosis in systemic lupus erythematosus: relation to the presence of circulating anticoagulants. Arch Intern Med 1985;145:1389–1395.

11. Parke AL, Wilson D, Maier D. The prevalence of antiphospholipid antibodies in women with recurrent spontaneous abortion, women with successful pregnancies and women who have never been pregnant. Arthritis Rheum 1991;34:1231–1235.

SCLERODERMA

Progressive systemic sclerosis (scleroderma) is a disease characterized by excessive skin thickening and internal organ fibrosis that can lead to dysphagia, gastrointestinal hypomotility, pulmonary fibrosis, cardiac abnormalities, hypertension, and renal failure. Over 90% of patients suffer from Raynaud's phenomenon. Histologically, there is an excessive deposition of collagen and obliteration of capillaries. The disease may present with evidence of inflammation, and there are overlap syndromes suggesting autoimmunity (CREST syndrome). A variety of autoantibodies may be present, including the scleroderma antibody (SCL-70), which is found in 20 to 60% of patients.

In an uncontrolled trial, TPE in combination with prednisone and cyclophosphamide was reported to produce substantial clinical improvement in 14 of 15 patients (1). **TPE prescription involved a one plasma volume exchange performed weekly for up to 10 exchanges and thereafter at 1- to 4-week intervals.** In a preliminary report of a controlled trial, 16 patients were randomized to receive no TPE, TPE alone, or TPE with lymphoplasmapheresis (2). TPE involving 50 mL/kg of plasma was performed 21 times over 3 months. Statistically significant improvement was found in both treatment groups compared with control subjects and was manifest in Rodman's skin score, physical therapy assessment, and global assessment. Unfortunately, there seems to be no formal publication of the final results of this study. In another controlled trial, in which most patients received one or two TPE treatments, there was objective improvement in the frequency of Raynaud's attacks and digital ulcer healing but no consistent objective improvement; some patients receiving "placebo" TPE had similar improvements as those treated with actual exchanges (3). In another report, a series of TPE treatments was attempted in seven patients (4). In three patients, treatment was discontinued because of insufficient vascular access. Between 8 and 20 TPE treatments were performed in the remaining four patients. Of these, only one patient, with an associated progressive myositis, noted benefit of articular and cutaneous symptoms. Recently, photopheresis was evaluated in a large, multicenter, controlled trial with *d*-penicillamine and was found to yield improved results in terms of skin severity score after 6 months of follow-up (5). In 1993, a review of the available literature concluded that TPE should be reserved for patients with active and rapidly progressive disease, progressive visceral involvement, or severe Raynaud's phenomenon (see Raynaud's Disease, below) (6). These reviewers recommended that **TPE should be performed with lymphoplasmapheresis on an every other day schedule. TPE should be with one plasma volume exchanges and lymphoplasmapheresis should remove 5×10^9 lymphocytes.** Vascular access may be difficult to obtain and usually requires central venous catheterization. Concomitant calcium replacement may be useful to decrease effects of citrate-induced hypocalcemia.

Recently, two separate reports described the coexistence of scleroderma and a particular type of normotensive normoreninemic renal disease (i.e., not compatible with scleroderma renal crises) in which the patients were positive for antineutrophil cytoplasmic autoantibodies (ANCA), which have been commonly associated with certain vasculitides such as Wegener's granulomatosis and periarteritis nodosa (7,8). In both reports, TPE seemed to offer clinical benefit. Endo et al. (7) evaluated 100 consecutive patients with scleroderma for the presence of ANCA. They found six patients (6%) to be positive for antimyeloperoxidase antibodies, a subset of the ANCAs. All six patients developed rapidly progressive renal failure with normotension and normal plasma renin levels (7). Pulmonary hemorrhage, anemia, and thrombocytopenia were associated morbidities. Other autoantibodies found in some patients included anti-nRNP, anti-DNA, anti-Sm, and LE cell antibodies. Outcome was poor except for one patient treated with plasmapheresis and cyclophosphamide. A similar patient was reported by Omote et al (8) in whom myeloperoxidase-specific ANCA was associated with a renal biopsy revealing a necrotizing crescentic glomerulonephritis (pauci-immune type) (see Rapidly Progressive Glomerulonephritis, Chap. 12). Methylprednisolone pulse therapy followed by prednisolone and mizoribine did not suppress the progression of renal failure. Double-filtration plasmapheresis effectively removed the myeloperoxidase-specific ANCA, and the authors concluded that it prevented renal failure despite a relatively low dose of immunosuppressive medication.

In a situation similar with the above-noted ANCA-associated cases, Wach et al (9) reported on three patients with severe, localized scleroderma in whom there were elevated titers of antinuclear antibodies. Treatment was with plasmapheresis (10 to 12 procedures) and systemic steroids, and all three had improvement in cutaneous and joint lesions after 2 months of therapy.

REFERENCES

1. Dau PC, Kahaleh MB, Sagebiel RW. Plasmapheresis and immunosuppressive drug therapy in scleroderma. Arthritis Rheum 1981;24:1128–1136.
2. Weiner SR, Kono DH, Osterman HA. Preliminary report on a controlled trial of apheresis in the treatment of scleroderma. Arthritis Rheum 1987;30:S24. Abstract.
3. McCune M, Winkelmann RK, Osmundson PJ, Pineda AA. Plasma exchange: a controlled study of the effect in patients with Raynaud's phenomenon and scleroderma. J Clin Apheresis 1983;1:206–214.
4. Guillevin L, Leon A, Levy Y, Bletry O, Gayraud M, Andreu G, Godeau P. Treatment of progressive systemic sclerosis with plasma exchange. Seven cases. Int J Artif Organs 1983;6:315–318.
5. Rook AH, Freundlich B, Jegasothy BV, Perez MI, Barr WG, Jimenez SA, Rietschel RL, Wintroub B, Kahaleh MB, Varga J, et al. Treatment of systemic sclerosis with extracorporeal photochemotherapy. Arch Dermatol 1992;128:337–346.

6. Kiprov DD, Strauss RG, Ciavarella D, Gilcher RO, Kasprisin DO, Klein HG, McLeod BC. Management of autoimmune disorders. J Clin Apheresis 1993;8:195–210.
7. Endo H, Hosono T, Kondo H. Antineutrophil cytoplasmic autoantibodies in 6 patients with renal failure and systemic sclerosis. J Rheumatol 1994;21:864–870.
8. Omote A, Muramatsu M, Sugimoto Y, Hosono S, Murakami R, Tanaka H, Watanabe Y, Sano H, Kato K. Myeloperoxidase-specific anti-neutrophil cytoplasmic autoantibodies-related scleroderma renal crisis treated with double-filtration plasmapheresis. Intern Med 1997;36:508–513.
9. Wach F, Ullrich H, Schmitz G, Landthaler M, Hein R. Treatment of severe localized scleroderma by plasmapheresis—report of three cases. Br J Dermatol 1995;133:605–609.

RHEUMATOID ARTHRITIS AND RHEUMATOID VASCULITIS

Rheumatoid arthritis is a chronic, systemic, inflammatory disease of unknown etiology in which destructive joint inflammation is a major distinguishing feature. Other systemic symptoms include malaise, fever, weight loss, and morning stiffness. Extra-articular manifestations include subcutaneous nodules, pleural effusion, pericarditis, lymphadenopathy, splenomegaly, and vasculitis. Serologic positivity for rheumatoid factor is usually present and supports an inflammatory pathogenesis.

In 1977, Paulus et al (1) demonstrated that lymphocyte depletion via a surgically created fistula in the thoracic duct was capable of decreasing the number of tender joints and decreasing the duration of morning stiffness in patients with rheumatoid arthritis. Subsequently, two randomized controlled studies using lymphapheresis as a means of lymphocyte depletion demonstrated similar benefit in reducing articular involvement (2,3), whereas a third trial of plasmapheresis without lymphocyte depletion demonstrated no benefit (4) (Table 11-2). Combining the results from these three randomized trials, one can conclude that plasmapheresis alone is not effective in chronic rheumatoid arthritis and that the relative value of lymphocytapheresis and lymphoplasmapheresis cannot be assessed, but the antirheumatic effect is relatively rapid in onset (1 to 2 weeks) with approximately 40 to 50% of patients having marked improvement for up to 3 months. Despite a documented, albeit modest, medical benefit, the use of lymphocytapheresis

Table 11-2. Lymphopheresis and Plasmapheresis in Rheumatoid Arthritis

Study	Procedure	Results
Paulus et al 1997 (Arthritis Rheum)	Lymphocyte depletion via thoracic duct	Nine patients with decreased number of tender joints and reduced duration of morning stiffness
Karsh et al 1981 (Arthritis Rheum)	Lymphapheresis randomized trial with sham procedure	Six patients treated had reduction in number of active swollen joints and graded articular index
Wallace et al 1982 (N Engl J Med)	Lymphoplasmapheresis double-blind controlled with sham procedure	Fourteen patients randomized; 7 treated had reduction in graded articular index
Dwosh et al 1983 (N Engl J Med)	Plasmapheresis controlled double-blind crossover trial	Twenty-six patients randomized. Despite biochemical improvement, no clinical improvement

for rheumatoid arthritis has been limited by its costs and inconvenience.

Given these constraints, Hamberger et al (5) suggested a limited set of conditions wherein the use of lymphocytapheresis or lymphoplasmapheresis for chronic rheumatoid arthritis could be justified. These would include continued active synovitis failing to respond to conventional and cytotoxic drug therapy, the concomitant administration of slow-acting antirheumatics, and a preset limit of nine treatments if there is no response.

Rheumatoid Vasculitis

Although TPE without lymphocyte depletion is not efficacious in the management of chronic rheumatoid arthritis, TPE may be useful in the treatment of rheumatoid-associated vasculitis, hyperviscosity, or peripheral neuropathy (6). Four reports described rapid clinical improvement in the management of patients with **severe necrotizing rheumatoid vasculitis**, with clinical resolution and healing of ulcerations concomitant with the lowering of high titers of circulating immune complexes (7–10). An early report related success in three of four patients, but the exchange volumes were not adequately detailed (7). In a subsequent paper describing success in two patients, treatment prescription was initiated with **two to three TPE treatments per week, gradually reducing treatment frequency for 6 to 9 weeks** (8). A similar approach resulted in clinical improvement in three patients after **a series of three 2-liter exchanges** (9). The largest series reported at least some success in seven of nine patients, but the exchange volumes were very limited (0.5 to 1.6 L/day). The best outcomes were in patients receiving a prolonged course (up to 38 treatments) (10). On a technical note, selective removal of circulating immune complexes in rheumatoid arthritis can be achieved with membrane filtration and cryogelation (11).

Patients with hyperviscosity syndrome should be treated as described in the section on hyperviscosity (see Chap. 8). Patients with peripheral neuropathy who have no other evidence for vasculitis may respond to the same regimen recommended for chronic inflammatory demyelinating polyneuropathy (see Chap. 7).

REFERENCES

1. Paulus HE, Machleder HI, Levine S, Yu DT, MacDonald NS. Lymphocyte involvement in rheumatoid arthritis. Arthritis Rheum 1977;20:1249–1262.
2. Karsh J, Klippel JH, Plotz PH, Decker JL, Wright DG, Flye MW. Lymphapheresis in rheumatoid arthritis: a randomized trial. Arthritis Rheum 1981;24:867–873.
3. Wallace DJ, Goldfinger D, Lowe C, Nichols S, Weiner J, Brachman M, Klinenberg JR. Double blind sham controlled trial of lymphoplasmapheresis versus sham pheresis in rheumatoid arthritis. N Engl J Med 1982;306:1406–1410.
4. Dwosh IL, Giles AR, Ford PM, Pater JL, Anastassiades TP and the Queen's University Plasmapheresis Study Group. Plasmapheresis therapy in rheumatoid arthritis: a controlled, double blind, crossover trial. N Engl J Med 1983;308:1124–1129.
5. Hamberger MI, Bennett RS, Kaell A. Apheresis in the treatment of rheumatoid arthritis. In: Pinada AA, Valbonesis M, Diggs JC, eds. Therapeutic hemapheresis. Milan, Italy: Wichtig Editore, 1986:77–82.

6. Kiprov DD, Strauss RG, Ciavarella D, Gilcher RO, Kasprisin DO, Klein HG, McLeod BC. Management of autoimmune disorders. J Clin Apheresis 1993;8:195–210.
7. Goldman JA, Casey HL, McIlwain H, Kirby J, Wilson Jr CH, Miller SB. Limited plasmapheresis in rheumatoid arthritis with vasculitis. Arthritis Rheum 1979;22:1146–1150.
8. Calabrese LH, Clough JD, Krakauer RS, Hoeltge GA. Plasmapheresis therapy of immunologic disease: report of nine cases and review of the literature. Cleve Clin Q 1980;47:53–72.
9. Brubaker DB, Winkelstein A. Plasma exchange in rheumatoid vasculitis. Vox Sang 1981;41:295–301.
10. Scott DGI, Bacon PA, Bothamley JE, Allen C, Elson CJ, Wallington TB. Plasma exchange in rheumatoid vasculitis. J Rheumatol 1981;8:433–439.
11. Krakauer RS, Asanuma Y, Sawicki I, Calabrese L, Malchesky P, Nose Y. Circulating immune complexes in rheumatoid arthritis: selective removal by cryogelation with membrane filtration. Arch Intern Med 1982;142:395–397.

VASCULITIS

Systemic vasculitis refers to a heterogenous group of disorders in which there is generalized inflammation of the blood vessels. Several categorizations have been proposed involving the size of the affected vessels and the presence or absence of granulomas. Included in this broad category are diseases such as polyarteritis nodosa, Wegener's granulomatosis, Churg-Strauss syndrome (CSS), microscopic polyarteritis, giant cell arteritis, and Takayasu's disease. Vasculitis may also occur as an expression of other systemic diseases such as SLE, rheumatoid arthritis, cryoglobulinemia, Behcet's syndrome, Henoch-Schönlein purpura, and Kawasaki disease.

Originally thought to be primarily a result of immune complex deposition (1), it is now well established that other autoimmune phenomena may be at play. Of particular note is the identification of ANCA, which has been shown to be associated with Wegener's granulomatosis, polyarteritis, and other systemic vasculitides.

Because these vasculitides often have a clinical expression that is dominated by a rapidly progressive glomerulonephritis (RPGN), many studies attempting to determine the usefulness of TPE have involved the treatment of glomerulonephritis and have been outlined in this book in the appropriate sections, including those on

SLE, IgA nephritis (Henoch-Schönlein purpura), cryoglobulinemia, and RPGN (Wegener's granulomatosis and other ANCA-associated diseases). The vasculitis associated with rheumatoid arthritis was covered in the last section. In this section, vasculitides not covered in these alternate sections are reviewed.

In an uncontrolled series reported from the National Institutes of Health, patients with severe systemic vasculitis associated with **Sjögren's syndrome** responded dramatically to TPE, with or without the addition of cyclophosphamide (2). **Prescription was with daily 3-liter exchanges for 1 to 2 weeks followed by alternate-day exchanges for up to a few weeks.** In another study, **polyarteritis nodosa (PN) associated with hepatitis B infection** was successfully treated with vidarabine and TPE (3). **During the first 3 weeks of treatment, 14 TPE treatments were performed, followed by three sessions per week for 2 weeks and then two sessions per week for 2 weeks.** Vidarabine was given by continuous infusion at 15 mg/kg/day for 7 days and then 7.5 mg/kg/day for 14 days. During subsequent weeks, TPE was performed once or twice a week. In 18 of 25 patients, the treatment was effective. Although unsubstantiated by a randomized controlled trial, this type of antiviral/TPE approach is particularly appealing for hepatitis B–associated PN because it avoids the use of steroids or immunosuppressive agents that may facilitate viral replication and the development of a chronic hepatitis B virus infection. A more recent study by the same authors replaced vidarabine with interferon alfa, an equally appealing approach (4,5).

In contrast to their results with hepatitis B–associated PN, these same authors conducted a prospective, randomized, multicenter trial in which 62 patients were randomly assigned to receive either prednisone plus cyclophosphamide or prednisone plus cyclophosphamide and plasma exchanges as first-line treatment for **severe PN or CSS. Patients with hepatitis B–associated PN were excluded.** They found no significant difference between the 5-year cumulative survival rates of the two groups and concluded that the addition of TPE to prednisone and pulse cyclophosphamide was not a superior treatment and should not be systematically proposed for the initial treatment of severe PN or CSS (6). A lack of particular benefit of TPE was also noted in a subsequent meta-analysis of those patients who presented with glomerulonephritis (7).

Thus, based on the outcome of a large cohort of patients with either **PN or CSS**, TPE added to steroids and cyclophosphamide was not found to be superior to steroids and cyclophosphamide alone, even in those patients presenting with glomerulonephritis. This is in contrast to the conclusions of the same authors regarding **hepatitis B–related PN**, in which TPE combined with antiviral therapy was found to be a useful protocol, especially because it did not require the use of steroids or immunosuppressive agents, which are considered undesirable in patients with latent viral disease.

REFERENCES

1. Lockwood CM, Worlledge S, Nicholas A, Cotton C, Peters DK. Reversal of impaired splenic function in patients with nephritis or vasculitis (or both) by plasma exchange. N Engl J Med 1979;300:524–530.
2. Fauci AS, Leavitt RY. Systemic vasculitis. In: Liechtenstein LM, Fauci AS, eds. Current therapy in allergy, immunology and rheumatology. Toronto: B. C. Decker, 1988:149–154.
3. Guillevin L, the Cooperative Study Group for the Study of Polyarteritis Nodosa. Treatment of polyarteritis nodosa and Churg-Strauss angiitis: indications of plasma exchange. Results of three prospective trials in 162 patients. In: Rock G, ed. Apheresis. New York: Wiley-Liss, 1990:321–325.
4. Guillevin L, Lhote F, Sauvaget F, Deblois P, Rossi F, Levallois D, Pourrat J, Christoforov B, Trepo C. Treatment of polyarteritis nodosa related hepatitis B virus with interferon-alpha and plasma exchanges. Ann Rheum Dis 1994;53:334–337.
5. Guillevin L, Lhote F, Cohen P, Sauvaget F, Jarrousse B, Lortholary O, Noel LH, Trepo C. Polyarteritis nodosa related to hepatitis B virus: a prospective study with long-term observation of 41 patients. Medicine 1995;74:238–253.
6. Guillevin L, Lhote F, Cohen P, Jarrousse B, Lortholary O, Genereau T, Leon A, Bussel A. Corticosteroids plus pulse cyclophosphamide and plasma exchanges versus corticosteroids plus pulse cyclophosphamide alone in the treatment of polyarteritis nodosa and Churg-Strauss syndrome patients with factors predicting poor prognosis. A prospective, randomized trial in sixty-two patients. Arthritis Rheum 1995;38:1638–1645.
7. Guillevin L, Cevallos R, Durand-Gasselin B, Lhote F, Jarrousse B, Callard P. Treatment of glomerulonephritis in microscopic polyangiitis and Churg-Strauss syndrome. Indications of plasma

exchanges, meta-analysis of 2 randomized studies on 140 patients, 32 with glomerulonephritis. Ann Med Interne (Paris) 1997;148:198–204.

POLYMYOSITIS AND DERMATOMYOSITIS

Polymyositis and dermatomyositis are often characterized as idiopathic inflammatory myopathies. Clinical symptoms include proximal and symmetric muscle weakness and muscle inflammation. In dermatomyositis, a skin rash may precede the myopathy. Creatine kinase levels are often elevated. Activated T and B lymphocytes and the presence of autoantibodies suggest an autoimmune etiology. In dermatomyositis, complement deposition in muscle capillaries precedes damage to capillaries and muscle, suggesting a disorder of humoral immunity and the possibility of benefit from TPE. Early uncontrolled trials and case reports suggested that plasma exchange or leukapheresis (as a means of removing activated lymphocytes) can improve the clinical course and histologic appearance of these diseases (1–4). More recently, a randomized controlled trial comparing either leukapheresis or TPE with sham apheresis reported no obvious benefit to either of these therapies (5). A review of the available evidence has concluded that TPE should be limited to clinical trials or as an adjunct to immunosuppressive therapy for acute disease (6).

Keeping in compliance with the previous recommendation, a recent report described a case of severe juvenile dermatomyositis with bowel vasculitis and pancreatitis in which improvement was obtained with a combination of TPE and immunosuppression (7).

REFERENCES

1. Brewer EJ, Giannini EH, Rossen RD, Patten B, Barkley E. Plasma exchange therapy of a childhood onset dermatomyositis patient. Arthritis Rheum 1980;23:509–513.
2. Dau PC. Plasmapheresis in idiopathic inflammatory myopathy: experience with 35 patients. Arch Neurol 1981;38:544–552.
3. Clarke CR, Dyall-Smith DJ, Mackay IR, Emery P, Jennens ID, Becker G. Plasma exchange in dermatomyositis/polymyositis: beneficial effects in three cases. J Clin Lab Immunol 1998; 27:149–152.

4. Bennington JL, Dau PC. Patients with polymyositis and dermatomyositis who undergo plasmapheresis therapy: pathologic findings. Arch Neurol 1981;38:553–560.
5. Miller FW, Leitman SF, Cronin ME, Hicks JE, Leff RL, Wesley R, Fraser DD, Dalakas M, Plotz PH. Controlled trial of plasma exchange and leukapheresis in polymyositis and dermatomyositis. N Engl J Med 1992;326:1380–1384.
6. Ciavarella D, Wuest D, Strauss RG, Gilcher RO, Kasprisin DO, Kiprov DD, Klein HG, McLeod BC. Management of neurologic disorders. J Clin Apheresis 1993;8:242–257.
7. See Y, Martin K, Rooney M, Woo P. Severe juvenile dermatomyositis complicated by pancreatitis. Br J Rheumatol 1997;36: 912–916.

RAYNAUD'S DISEASE

In 1978, Tolpos et al (1) reported on an uncontrolled trial involving five patients with severe treatment-resistant Raynaud's disease for whom TPE produced a striking improvement. Ultrasonic velocimetry showed that segments of digital arteries that had been thought to be permanently occluded became patent and remained patent after plasmapheresis. Subsequently, O'Reilly et al (2) published a study in which 27 patients with Raynaud's syndrome were randomized to receive either placebo, heparin, or TPE. TPE prescription was **2 to 2.5 L/wk for 4 weeks**. Evaluation of study groups was by Doppler ultrasound assessment of digital vessels. Neither placebo nor heparin had any effect on the patency of the digital vessels or on the patients' symptoms, whereas the TPE-treated group had improvement in both symptoms and vessel patency. In seven of eight TPE-treated patients, improvement was maintained for 6 months. Possible mechanisms by which TPE could be a successful treatment for Raynaud's disease were reviewed by Hamilton et al (3) and include reduction in viscosity, not only by removal of fibrinogen but by improvement in red blood cell deformability and reduction in immunoglobulins and immune complexes. Of note is that in the controlled study of O'Reilly et al, viscosity remained reduced for up to 6 months.

REFERENCES

1. Talpos G, White JM, Horrocks M, Cotton LT. Plasmapheresis in Raynaud's disease. Lancet 1978;1:416–417.

2. O'Reilly MJG, Talpos G, Roberts VC. Controlled trial of plasma exchange in treatment of Raynaud's syndrome. Br Med J 1979;1:1113–1115.
3. Hamilton WAP, O'Reilly MJG, Dodds AJ. Plasma exchange in Raynaud's phenomenon. Lancet 1980;2:475. Letter.

Renal Disease

12

Anti-GBM Antibody-Mediated Disease (Goodpasture's Syndrome)   180
Rapidly Progressive Glomerulonephritis   182
Renal Failure in Multiple Myeloma   186
IgA Nephropathy and Henoch-Schönlein Purpura   190
    Henoch-Schönlein Purpura   191
Focal Segmental Glomerulosclerosis: Recurrence Post-Transplant   192
Renal Allograft Rejection   193
The Transplant Candidate with Cytotoxic Antibodies   195

Most glomerulonephritides are immunologically based, with clear evidence of either linear anti–glomerular basement membrane (GBM) deposition or granular immune complex deposition. Even those glomerulonephritides that were previously considered to be "pauci-immune," with no obvious immunoglobulin deposition in the glomerulus, are now known to be associated with an antineutrophil cytoplasmic antibody (ANCA). Thus, it is not surprising that many investigators attempted to treat these disorders with plasma exchange (1–3). A role for therapeutic plasma exchange (TPE) as a means of steroid "sparing" or in limiting the use of immunosuppressive medication is particularly appealing. TPE is also useful for the removal of nephrotoxic light chains in the presence of the "cast nephropathy" associated with multiple myeloma.

"Primary" renal indications for TPE are listed in Table 12-1. Notably absent from this list are the nephritides associated with certain systemic diseases. Indications for TPE in the management of the renal diseases associated with **systemic lupus erythematosus (SLE), the antiphospholid antibody syndrome (lupus anticoagulant), and the systemic vasculitides** are presented in Chapter 11. TPE treatments for the nephritides associ-

Table 12-1. Renal Indications for TPE

	Reference and Year		
	1 1986	2 1993	3 1994
	Rating		
Renal disease			
Goodpasture's syndrome	I	I	I
Rapidly progressive glomerulonephritis	I	II	II
Multiple myeloma, "cast nephropathy"	II	II	nl
Henoch-Schönlein purpura/IgA nephropathy	II	nl	nl
Focal segmental glomerulosclerosis: recurrence post-transplant	nl	nl	nl
Renal allograft rejection	II	IV	IV
Removal of cytotoxic antibodies in the transplant candidate	nl	nl	nl

Rating: I, standard therapy, acceptable but not mandatory; II, available evidence tends to favor efficacy: conventional therapy usually tried first; III, inadequately tested at this time; IV, no demonstrated value in controlled trials. nl, not listed.
REFERENCES: 1. American Medical Association Council on Scientific Affairs. Current status of therapeutic plasmapheresis. JAMA 1985;253:819–825.
2. Strauss RG, Ciavarella D, Gilcher RO, Kasprisin DO, Kiprov DD, Klein HG, McLeod BC. An overview of current management. J Clin Apheresis 1993;8:189–194.
3. Leitman SF, Ciavarella D, McLeod B, Owen H, Price T, Sniecinski I. Guidelines for therapeutic hemapheresis. Bethesda, MD: American Association of Blood Banks, revised 1994.

ated with **cryoglobulinemia and the hemolytic uremic syndrome** are presented in Chapter 8. Multiple myeloma is listed in this chapter because light chain–induced cast nephropathy represents the major indication for TPE in this disorder.

REFERENCES

1. Sakellariou G. Plasmapheresis as a therapy in specific forms of acute renal failure. Nephrol Dial Transplant 1994;9(suppl 4):210–218.
2. Madore F, Lazarus JM, Brady HR. Therapeutic plasma exchange in renal disease. J Am Soc Nephrol 1996;7:367–386.
3. Kaplan AA. Therapeutic plasma exchange for renal disease. Semin Dial 1996;9:61–70.

ANTI-GBM ANTIBODY-MEDIATED DISEASE (GOODPASTURE'S SYNDROME)

There has been only one randomized controlled study of plasma exchange as an adjunct to immunosuppressive therapy for anti-GBM antibody-mediated glomerulonephritis. This study used a relatively inefficient TPE prescription (once every 3 days as opposed to daily treatments) and was unequally randomized, with the non-TPE group having a more severe presentation of renal disease (a greater amount of interstitial fibrosis and tubular atrophy) (1). Nonetheless, the results of this study and that of other nonrandomized or case-controlled studies are generally in agreement that plasma exchange is useful in providing a more rapid decline in the serum levels of anti-GBM antibody, a lower post-treatment serum creatinine level, and a decreased incidence of end-stage renal disease (ESRD) (2–5). TPE has also been found to have a beneficial effect on the course of severe pulmonary hemorrhage (2,6). It should be noted, however, that the best correlation with a positive renal outcome is the initiation of therapy before the onset of severe renal impairment. Avoidance of ESRD is uncommon if treatment is begun after serum creatinine exceeds 7 mg/dL. Nonetheless, even patients presenting with severe renal impairment have responded to therapy if the presentation is very acute (2,7,8) or there are signs of associated vasculitis and positivity for ANCA (7,9). In a retrospective study of 889 cases of rapidly progressive glomerulonephritis (see below), 47 (5%) were positive only for anti-GBM antibodies, 246 (28%) were positive only for ANCA, and 20 (2%) had both (9). Analyzed from a different perspective, there were 67 patients positive for anti-GBM antibodies in whom 20 (30%) were also positive for ANCA.

TPE is prescribed to provide a rapid lowering of the anti-GBM antibody and possibly as a means of reducing the serum concentrations of other potentially detrimental inflammatory mediators, such as complement. An immunosuppressive regimen with steroids, cyclophosphamide, or azathioprine is essential as a means of slowing the production of the anti-GBM antibody and decreasing the inflammatory response.

The recommended plasmapheresis prescription is 14 daily 4-liter exchanges. In general, albumin can be used as the replacement fluid (see below). The patient should be reassessed at the end of this 2-week regimen. Further plasmapheresis may be unnecessary if serum creatinine levels have decreased and there is a marked decline in serum anti-GBM antibody titers. In contrast, **continued apheresis may be required if antibody titers are still elevated**, and **certain patients have required as many as 25 treatments** for successful lowering of the serum antibody titers (3).

Such an intensive replacement of plasma with albumin will yield a depletion coagulopathy as evident by marked elevations of the prothrombin times and partial thromboplastin times. There is also a virtual elimination of all serum immunoglobulins. Thus, the patient with a recent renal biopsy or with significant pulmonary hemorrhage may benefit from a partial replacement with fresh frozen plasma (FFP). In our experience, depletion coagulopathy can be partially corrected by substituting 1 to 2 liters of FFP as the replacement fluid toward the end of the procedure (10) (each unit of FFP is approximately 200 to 250 mL) (see Chap. 4, Fig. 4-1). One potential complication with FFP (14% citrate by volume) is the development of metabolic alkalosis because the metabolism of citrate will produce bicarbonate, the excretion of which may be limited by concurrent renal failure. This alkalosis may also occur if citrate is used as the anticoagulant during the procedure, as is commonly done with centrifugal apheresis equipment (11).

The apheresis-induced immunoglobulin deficiency may predispose to or exacerbate an intercurrent infection. If the infection is severe, a single infusion of immunoglobulin (100 to 400 mg/kg) will partially replenish antibody levels that were reduced by the exchanges (10), keeping in mind that continued apheresis will eventually deplete these infused immunoglobulins.

Although plasma exchange therapy may be discontinued once anti-GBM antibody titers have been lowered, immunosuppressive therapy is generally continued for 6 to 12 months, after which there is often a spontaneous cessation of autoantibody formation. Late recurrences have been documented (12).

REFERENCES

1. Johnson JP, Moore JJ, Austin H III, Balow JE, Antonovych TT, Wilson CB. Therapy of anti glomerular basement membrane disease: analysis of prognostic significance of clinical, pathologic and treatment factors. Medicine 1985;64:219–227.
2. Savage CO, Pusey CD, Bowman C, Rees AJ, Lockwood CM. Antiglomerular basement membrane antibody-mediated

disease in the British Isles 1980–4. Br Med J 1986;292:301–304.

3. Simpson IJ, Doak PB, Williams LC, Blacklock HA, Hill RS, Teague CA, Herdson PB, Wilson CB. Plasma exchange in Goodpasture's syndrome. Am J Nephrol 1982;2:301–311.

4. Lockwood CM, Rees AJ, Pearson TA, Evans DJ, Peters DK, Wilson CB. Immunosuppression and plasma exchange in the treatment of Goodpasture's syndrome. Lancet 1976;1:711–714.

5. Madore F, Lazarus JM, Brady HR. Therapeutic plasma exchange in renal disease. J Am Soc Nephrol 1996;7:367–386.

6. McCarthy LJ, Cotton J, Danielson C, Graves V, Bergstein J. Goodpasture's syndrome in childhood: treatment with plasmapheresis and immunosuppression. J Clin Apheresis 1994;9:116–119.

7. Maxwell AP, Nelson WE, Hill CM. Reversal of renal failure in nephritis associated with antibodies to glomerular basement membrane. Br Med J 1988;297:333–334.

8. Fort J, Espinel E, Rogriquez JA, Curull V, Madrenas J, Piera L. Partial recovery of renal function in an oligoanuric patient affected with Goodpasture's syndrome after treatment with steroids, immunosuppressives and plasmapheresis. Clin Nephrol 1984;22:211–212. Letter.

9. Jayne DRW, Marshall PD, Jones SJ, Lockwood CM. Autoantibodies to GBM and neutrophil cytoplasm in rapidly progressive glomerulonephritis. Kidney Int 1990;37:965–970.

10. Mokrzycki MH, Kaplan AA. Therapeutic plasma exchange: complications and management. Am J Kidney Dis 1994;23:817–827.

11. Pearl RG, Rosenthal MH. Metabolic alkalosis due to plasmapheresis. Am J Med 1985;79:391–393.

12. Klasa RJ, Abboud RT, Ballon HS, Grossman L. Goodpasture's syndrome: recurrence after a five-year remission. Am J Med 1988;84:751–755.

RAPIDLY PROGRESSIVE GLOMERULONEPHRITIS (NOT ASSOCIATED WITH ANTI-GBM ANTIBODY)

With the identification of the ANCA-associated pauci-immune glomerulonephritides, most patients with rapidly progressive glomerulonephritis (RPGN) can be classified as to their etiology, and the diagnosis of "idiopathic" RPGN is becoming rare (1). Thus, most patients with this diagnosis can be identified as having anti-

GBM disease, ANCA-associated disease, or a variety of well-defined immune complex deposition diseases such as lupus, IgA, or cryoglobulinemic-associated glomerulonephritides. In a retrospective study of 889 cases of RPGN, Jayne et al (2) reported that 47 (5%) were positive only for anti–GBM antibodies, 246 (28%) were positive only for ANCA, and 20 (2%) had both, whereas 576 (65%) had neither and probably had one of the systemic diseases listed above (SLE, IgA, cryoglobulinemia, etc.). Considering our new-found ability to classify these nephritides, the previous studies evaluating the potential benefit of TPE for idiopathic RPGN are difficult to evaluate. In any event, because most pauci-immune glomerulonephritides are now known to be ANCA associated, one might extrapolate the available data accordingly.

Treatment of the various types of RPGN often involves steroids and some form of immunosuppressive regimen. TPE has been investigated as a means to rapidly remove pathogenic autoantibodies, immune complexes, and other inflammatory mediators such as complement and fibrinogen (3). In general, TPE has been found to be a relatively safe but costly addition to more conventional treatment regimens. This added expense should be viewed in the context of the eventual long-term cost of maintenance dialysis for those patients who are not successfully treated and whose outcome will terminate with end stage renal disease (ESRD).

Despite favorable uncontrolled reports (4–6), the results of four randomized, controlled studies failed to demonstrate a generalized benefit for TPE in the treatment of non-anti-GBM-associated RPGN when added to standard immunosuppressive therapy (7–10). Nonetheless, in all of these studies, subset analysis reveals that TPE was found to be beneficial for those patients presenting with severe disease or dialysis dependency (Table 12-2) (11). In one study in which this issue was specifically addressed, Pusey et al (9) randomized 48 patients with crescentic glomerulonephritis in whom anti-GBM disease and other well-defined vasculitides (SLE and Henoch-Schönlein purpura) were excluded. Although the patients were not tested for ANCA antibodies, the clinical diagnoses were that of Wegener's granulomatosis, microscopic polyarteritis, and idiopathic RPGN. In 25 patients, plasma exchange was initiated with **five 4-liter exchanges in the first week with a subsequent mean total of 9 treatments per patient (range, 5 to 25)**. Immunosuppressive treatment with prednisolone, cyclophosphamide, and azathioprine was administered to all 48 patients. Results revealed no outcome difference in those patients

Table 12-2. Controlled Trials of TPE for Patients with Severe or Dialysis-Dependent RPGN[a]

	Index of Severity	TPE	No TPE
Mauri et al 1985 (7)	Creatinine > 9		
Initial creatinine		13.5 (6)	13.1 (5)
Creatinine after 3 yr		8.7[b]	13.4
Glockner et al 1988 (8)	Dialysis dependent		
Initial creatinine		7.4 (8)	9.2 (4)
Creatinine after 6 mo		1.7[b]	5.5
Pusey et al 1991 (9)	Dialysis dependent		
Initial no. of patients on dialysis		11	8
Patients off dialysis at 12 mo		10[c]	3
Cole et al 1992 (10)	Dialysis dependent		
Initial no. of patients on dialysis		4	7
Patients off dialysis at 12 mo		3	2

All studies had concomitant treatment with steroids and immunosuppressive agents. Values in parentheses are numbers of patients.
[a] Subset analysis, creatinine values in mg/dL.
[b] $p < 0.05$ with day 0.
[c] $p < 0.05$ TPE vs. no TPE.
SOURCE: Modified by permission from Kaplan AA. Therapeutic plasma exchange for the treatment of rapidly progressive glomerulonephritis (RPGN). Ther Apheresis 1997;1:255–259.

in whom treatment was initiated when serum creatinines were less than 500 µmol/L (5.8 mg/dL). Of those patients who were originally dialysis dependent, however, 10 of 11 receiving TPE recovered renal function, whereas only 3 of 8 in the non–TPE group recovered to a similar degree ($p = 0.04$). Thus, the results of this study and the three other controlled trials support the use of TPE in RPGN only in those patients presenting with severe renal failure or dialysis dependency. A recent review concluded that if TPE is used, **it should be performed at least four times during the first week, with 4-liter exchanges replaced with albumin** (12). Given the aggressive scheduling, partial replacement with FFP should be considered to mitigate postpheresis coagulopathy in the postbiopsy period or in the presence of pulmonary hemorrhage (see Chap. 4, Fig. 4-1).

It is of note that reserving TPE treatment for only those with severe disease is in sharp contrast to the general recommendation for treatment of anti-GBM-associated disease, in which there is strong evidence supporting the early initiation of treatment, before severe renal failure is present (see previous section).

Of interest is that all but one of the published TPE trials with non-anti-GBM-mediated RPGN were performed without randomization of patients by ANCA positivity or type. In the one trial that did assess this serology, only half the patients were tested and four of seven were ANCA positive in the non-TPE group, whereas six of seven were ANCA positive in the TPE group (13).

It has been suggested that a different method of plasmapheresis may be indicated in patients with hemoptysis. Most patients with Wegener's granulomatosis form IgG ANCA, but in a study of 24 consecutive patients with IgG ANCA-positive vasculitis, 8 were found to have IgM ANCA and 7 of these 8 presented with severe pulmonary hemorrhage (11). If the IgM antibodies are pathogenic, then a centrifugal method of plasma exchange may be preferred because standard membrane plasma separation may be less efficient in removing the large IgM-containing immune complexes (see Chap. 3, Fig. 3-3).

REFERENCES

1. Angangco R, Thiru S, Esnault VL, Short AK, Lockwood CM, Oliveira DBG. Does truly "idiopathic" crescentic glomerulonephritis exist? Nephrol Dial Transplant 1994;9:630–636.
2. Jayne DRW, Marshall PD, Jones SJ, Lockwood CM. Autoantibodies to GBM and neutrophil cytoplasm in rapidly progressive glomerulonephritis. Kidney Int 1990;37:965–970.
3. Glassock RJ. Intensive plasma exchange in crescentic glomerulonephritis: help or no help? Am J Kidney Dis 1992;20:270–275.
4. Lockwood CM, Rees AJ, Pinching AJ, Pussell B, Sweny P, Uff J, Peters DK. Plasma exchange and immunosuppression in the treatment of fulminating immune complex crescentic nephritis. Lancet 1977;1:63–67.
5. Kincaid-Smith P, D'Apice AJF. Plasmapheresis in rapidly progressive glomerulonephritis. Am J Med 1978;65:564–566.
6. Hind CRK, Paraskevakou H, Lockwood CM, Evans DJ, Peters DK, Rees AJ. Prognosis after immunosuppression of patients

with crescentic nephritis requiring dialysis. Lancet 1983;1:263–265.

7. Mauri JM, Gonzales MT, Poveda R, Seron D, Torras J, Andujar J, Andres E, Alsina J. Therapeutic plasma exchange in the treatment of rapidly progressive glomerulonephritis. Plasma Ther Transfus Technol 1985;6:587–591.

8. Glockner WM, Sieberth HG, Wichmann HE, Backes E, Bambauer R, Boesken WH, Bohle A, Daul A, Graben N, Keller F, Klehr U, Kohler H, Metz U, Schultz W, Thoenes W, Vlaho M. Plasma exchange and immunosuppression in rapidly progressive glomerulonephritis: a controlled multi-center study. Clin Nephrol 1988;29:1–8.

9. Pusey CD, Rees AJ, Evans DJ, Peters DK, Lockwood CM. Plasma exchange in focal necrotizing glomerulonephritis without anti-GBM antibodies. Kidney Int 1991;40:757–763.

10. Cole E, Cattran D, Magil A, Greenwood C, Churchill D, Sutton D, Clark W, Morrin P, Posen G, Bernstein K, Dyck R, and the Canadian Apheresis Study Group. A prospective randomized trial of plasma exchange as additive therapy in idiopathic crescentic glomerulonephritis. Am J Kidney Dis 1992;20:261–269.

11. Kaplan AA. Therapeutic plasma exchange for the treatment of rapidly progressive glomerulonephritis (RPGN). Ther Apheresis 1997;1:255–259.

12. Madore F, Lazarus JM, Brady HR. Therapeutic plasma exchange in renal disease. J Am Soc Nephrol 1996;7:367–386.

13. Esnault VL, Soleimani B, Keogan MT, Brownlee AA, Jayne DR, Lockwood CM. Association of IgM with IgG ANCA in patients presenting with pulmonary hemorrhage. Kidney Int 1992;41:1304–1310.

RENAL FAILURE IN MULTIPLE MYELOMA

Multiple myeloma is a malignant plasma cell dyscrasia with the autonomous growth of a single clone of plasma cells. Uncontrolled immunoglobulin secretion from this single clone yields the production of a monoclonal antibody. Disordered immunoglobulin synthesis is often associated with the overproduction of light chains, which may be toxic to renal tubules, resulting in renal failure. Nonetheless, renal failure is a relatively common problem in patients with multiple myeloma and may result from a variety of causes, including dehydration, hypercalcemia, hyperuricemia, pyelonephritis, plasma cell infiltration, amyloidosis, light chain deposition disease (1) (primarily a glomerular disease), and cast nephropathy, which is the result of the tubular-toxic effect of light chains and their tendency to obstruct the nephron lumen (2). It should be noted, therefore, that the recommended use of TPE for the reversal of myeloma-associated renal failure is only rational as a means of removing toxic light chains from the serum as a treatment for cast nephropathy.

After a reasonable diagnostic evaluation geared to rule out other common forms of myeloma-associated renal failure, including a therapeutic trial of hydration, patients with myeloma-associated renal failure and elevated *serum* levels of free light chains have a high likelihood of myeloma cast nephropathy. This can usually be detected as an M spike in the globulin region on serum protein electrophoresis. Concurrent urine protein electrophoresis should demonstrate a monoclonal spike in the same region (Fig. 12-1). Immunofixation should be used to confirm that the serum spike represents free light chains and not the complete immunoglobulin. Confirmation that the urine spike represents free light chains should also be confirmed by immunofixation because the standard Bence Jones test may produce both false negatives and false positives (3).

Once cast nephropathy is identified as the most likely cause for the renal failure, the rapid lowering of *serum* light chains by TPE, in conjunction with a proper antineoplastic regimen (usually a combination of steroids with melphalan or cyclophosphamide), has been demonstrated to provide a more likely return of renal function and a better overall survival. In a randomized controlled trial of 29 patients with mean pretreatment serum creatinine levels of 11 mg/dL, 13 of 15 patients treated with plasmapheresis (**3 to 4 liters of plasma exchanged on 5 consecutive days**) had substantial return of renal function (to a mean creatinine of 2.6 mg/dL) within 2 months, whereas improvement occurred in only 2 of 14 treated without plasmapheresis (4) (Table 12-3).

Well-established renal failure considered to be due to cast nephropathy may respond less dramatically, but a combination of TPE and chemotherapy has been successful if treatment is initiated before the onset of oligoanuria (5,6). Johnson et al (6) recommend the use of biopsy to determine the density of cast formation as a guide to the eventual response to TPE. If renal biopsy is performed and plasmapheresis initiated soon after, there is a potential risk of postbiopsy bleeding from apheresis-induced removal of coagulation

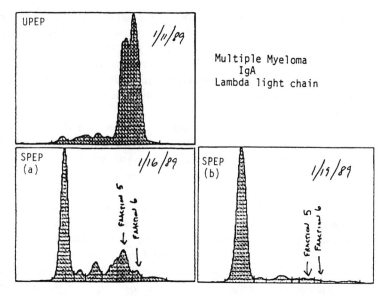

Figure 12-1. **Light chains in serum and urine in a case of biopsy-proven "cast nephropathy." Top left: Abnormal light chains noted on urine protein electrophoresis. Bottom left: Light chain "spike" found on the serum protein electrophoretic pattern during episode of renal failure. In general, light chains are freely filtered and are not normally found in appreciable amounts in the serum unless there is significant renal failure. Note that the light chain spike is found in the same position on both the urine and serum electrophoretic patterns. Bottom right: "flattening" of the serum protein electrophoretic pattern after four TPE treatments with albumin as the replacement fluid.**

factors, and partial replacement with FFP is recommended to attenuate the coagulopathy (see Chap. 4, Fig. 4-1).

If chemotherapy is successful in limiting new light chain synthesis, then a single prescription of five consecutive plasma exchanges may be sufficient (see Fig. 12-1). Further treatments may be necessary if there is continued light chain production. Wahlin et al (7) successfully used a prophylactic treatment prescription involving chemotherapy and **TPE three times weekly every 5 weeks** with comparison data suggesting substantially improved survival when compared with patients treated with chemotherapy alone. Having identified a given abnormal spike as a light chain by immunofixation, regular monitoring by serum protein electrophoresis is an easy means to detect recurrent light chain accumulation.

Table 12-3. Controlled Study of TPE for the Treatment of "Cast Nephropathy"

	Group 1 (TPE)	Group 2 (Control)
At onset		
Number of patients	15	14
Mean age (yr)	63	63
Kappa/lambda	9/6	8/6
Serum creatinine (mg/dL)	11.2	9.2
Number of patients requiring dialysis at onset	8	8
Short-term results		
Number of patients requiring dialysis	13	11
Number of patients interrupting dialysis	11	2*
Number of patients dying within 2 mo	1	5
Serum creatinine after 2 mo (mg/dL)	2.6	7.7*
Long-term results		
Number of patients alive after 18 mo	8	1*
Number of patients alive after 24 mo	7	1*
Number of patients alive after 32 mo	3	1*

*$p < 0.01$ between TPE- and non-TPE-treated patients.
SOURCE: Adapted from Zucchelli P, Pasquali S, Cagnali L, Ferrari G. Controlled plasma exchange trial in acute renal failure due to multiple myeloma. Kidney Int 1988;33:1175.

Although light chains are relatively small proteins (~20,000 Da), standard dialytic techniques are not capable of efficient light chain removal. In one study, net light chain removal in 50 liters of peritoneal dialysate was only 2 g, in contrast with the 17 g removed by one 5-liter plasma exchange (8). Standard "low flux" dialysis, with relatively "tight" membranes, is clearly incapable of substantial light chain removal, and the author's single attempt to document light chain removal by high-flux hemodialysis was unsuccessful (unpublished observation). Convection-based hemofiltration may be more effective but has yet to be evaluated as a means of light chain removal.

REFERENCES

1. Buxbaum JN, Chuba JV, Hellman GC, Solomon A, Gallo GR. Monoclonal immunoglobulin deposition disease: light chain and light and heavy chain deposition diseases and their relation to

light chain amyloidosis. Clinical features, immunopathology, and molecular analysis. Ann Intern Med 1990;112:455–464.

2. Solomon A, Weiss DT, Kattine AA. Nephrotoxic potential of Bence Jones proteins. N Engl J Med 1991;324:1845–1851.

3. Perry MC, Kyle RA. The clinical significance of Bence Jones proteinuria. Mayo Clin Proc 1975;50:234–238.

4. Zucchelli P, Pasquali S, Cagnoli L, Ferrari G. Controlled plasma exchange trial in acute renal failure due to multiple myeloma. Kidney Int 1988;33:1175–1189.

5. Misiani R, Tiraboschi G, Mingardi G, Mecca G. Management of myeloma kidney: an anti-light chain approach. Am J Kidney Dis 1987;10:28–33.

6. Johnson WJ, Kyle RA, Pineda AA, et al. Treatment of renal failure associated with multiple myeloma. Plasmapheresis, hemodialysis, and chemotherapy. Arch Intern Med 1990;150: 863–869.

7. Wahlin A, Lofvenberg E, Holm J. Improved survival in multiple myeloma with renal failure. Acta Med Scand 1987;221:205–209.

8. Russell JA, Fitzharris BM, Corringham R, et al. Plasma exchange v peritoneal dialysis for removing Bence Jones protein. Br Med J 1978;2:1397.

IgA NEPHROPATHY AND HENOCH-SCHÖNLEIN PURPURA

IgA nephropathy is the most common form of glomerulonephritis. Originally considered to be relatively benign, prolonged follow-up suggests that 30 to 35% of patients will progress to ESRD (1). Most patients will have a relatively indolent course, but about 10% will present with a rapidly progressive glomerulonephritis with exuberant crescent formation and an accelerated decline to irreversible renal failure. Henoch-Schönlein purpura has as its renal component a glomerular involvement that appears to be indistinguishable from the nonsystemic form of primary IgA nephropathy. The mesangial deposition of circulating IgA-containing immune complexes appears to be an integral factor in the disease process of both IgA nephropathy and the nephritis of Henoch-Schönlein purpura, but the actual pathogenesis is unclear and may involve a dysregulation of IgA synthesis. The removal of circulating IgA complexes by plasma exchange would appear to be an appealing therapeutic approach and in case reports and uncontrolled trials has been considered successful in the amelioration of both acute and chronically progressive disease (2–5). Nonetheless, the current availability of alternative treatment modalities, such as the use of fish oil and angiotensin-converting enzyme inhibitors (1), would appear to have eclipsed TPE as a treatment option for chronic progressive IgA nephropathy.

The potential usefulness of TPE as a treatment for acute disease remains unresolved. In one series, Hene and Kater (2) report a substantial decline in serum creatinine in two patients presenting with rapidly progressive disease in which plasma exchange was used without steroids or any other immunosuppressive treatment. Indeed, in a review of the literature, Coppo et al (3) list 7 case reports in which RPGN was successfully treated with TPE alone. In another report of acute fulminant disease, TPE was used in conjunction with cyclophosphamide and low-dose prednisone, achieving complete clinical remission (4). Although it could not be established that TPE played a significant role in the successful treatment of this patient, it was clear that the plasma exchange treatments were most responsible for the rapid lowering of circulating IgA immune complexes. More recently, in a rare case of alveolar hemorrhage associated with IgA nephropathy, TPE was reported to provide rapid improvement in the steroid-resistant nephritis (6). Thus, although there is no randomized controlled trial for evaluation, the currently available data suggest a possible beneficial effect of TPE in the treatment of IgA-associated RPGN. **A reasonable initial prescription would be to perform TPE thrice weekly for 3 weeks and then once weekly. Albumin can be used as the replacement fluid.**

Henoch-Schönlein Purpura

Although no formal series is available for assessment, single case reports suggested that TPE may also be of value in the management of nonrenal morbidities associated with Henoch-Schönlein purpura. Thus, TPE has been reported to be of value in the treatment of two patients with Henoch-Schönlein purpura and severe ileal or jejunal involvement (7,8) and in the management of a pregnant patient with suspected Henoch-Schönlein purpura (9).

REFERENCES

1. Galla JH. IgA nephropathy. Kidney Int 1995;47:377–387.
2. Hene RJ, Kater L. Plasmapheresis in nephritis associated with Henoch-Schönlein purpura and in primary IgA nephropathy. Plasma Ther Transfus Technol 1983;4:165–173.

3. Coppo R, Basolo B, Roccatello D, Piccoli G. Plasma exchange in primary IgA nephropathy and Henoch-Schönlein syndrome nephritis. Plasma Ther Transfus Technol 1985;6:705–723.

4. Coppo R, Basolo B, Giachino O, Roccatello D, Lajolo D, Mazzucco G, Amore A, Piccoli G. Plasmapheresis in a patient with rapidly progressive idiopathic IgA nephropathy: removal of IgA-containing circulating immune complexes and clinical recovery. Nephron 1985;40:488–490.

5. Nicholls K, Becker G, Walker R, Wright C, Kincaid-Smith P. Plasma exchange in progressive IgA nephropathy. J Clin Apheresis 1990;5:128–132.

6. Afessa B, Cowart RG, Koenig SM. Alveolar hemorrhage in IgA nephropathy treated with plasmapheresis. South Med J 1977; 90:237–239.

7. Gaskell H, Searle M, Dathan JR. Henoch-Schönlein purpura with severe ileal involvement responding to plasmapheresis. Int J Artif Organs 1985;8:163–164.

8. Morichau-Beauchant M, Touchard G, Maire P, Briaud M, Babin P, Alcalay D, Matuchansky C. Jejunal IgA and C3 deposition in adult Henoch-Schönlein purpura with severe intestinal manifestations. Gastroenterology 1982;82:1438–1442.

9. Joseph G, Holtman JS, Kosfeld RE, Blodgett WA, Liu YK. Pregnancy in Henoch-Schönlein purpura. Am J Obstet Gynecol 1987;157:911–912.

FOCAL SEGMENTAL GLOMERULOSCLEROSIS: RECURRENCE POST-TRANSPLANT

It has been estimated that 15 to 55% of all patients with ESRD secondary to focal segmental glomerular sclerosis (FSGS) have a rapid recurrence of proteinuria after renal transplantation. Recent studies suggest that some of these patients may have a circulating protein that is capable of increasing glomerular permeability to albumin. The protein has been characterized to have a molecular weight less than 100,000 Da and is therefore not an immunoglobulin (1). Nonetheless, a trial of immunoadsorption using a regenerating protein A column (ostensibly designed for the removal of three of four classes of IgG; see Immunoadsorbant Techniques, Chap. 3) was capable of transiently lowering the level of proteinuria in patients with recurrent FSGS after transplantation (1). Far more encouraging is a subsequent report in which standard plasma exchange was performed in patients soon after the recurrence of proteinuria in the immediate post-transplant period (2). Patients were treated with **plasma exchange for 3 consecutive days followed by every other day treatments for a total of nine exchanges. Each treatment consisted of the removal of 1.5 plasma volumes** with 5% albumin being used as the replacement fluid. Six of nine patients treated within 1 week of the onset of proteinuria had a mean reduction in protein excretion from 11.5 to 0.8 g/day, with at least one patient maintaining normal allograft histology for up to 27 months after treatment. Two patients relapsed and then responded to a repeat course of plasmapheresis. Two of the three nonresponders (as opposed to one of six responders) already had glomerular hyalinosis on renal biopsy. Based on these results, the authors concluded that plasma exchange is likely to be effective in the treatment of recurrent FSGS if treatment is initiated promptly after the initiation of proteinuria and there is no significant hyalinosis on preplasmapheresis biopsy.

REFERENCES

1. Dantal J, Bigot E, Bogers W, Testa A, Kriaa F, Jacques Y, Hurault de Ligny B, Niaudet P, Charpentier B, Soulillou JP. Effect of plasma protein adsorption on protein excretion in kidney-transplant recipients with recurrent nephrotic syndrome. N Engl J Med 1994;330:7–14.
2. Artero ML, Sharma R, Savin VJ, Vincenti F. Focal segmental glomerulosclerosis in renal transplants. Am J Kidney Dis 1994;23:574–581.

RENAL ALLOGRAFT REJECTION

The assumed role of cytotoxic antibodies as mediators of acute vascular rejection prompted several attempts to use plasma exchange as a means of enhancing antirejection therapy. Unfortunately, despite a rational and extensive therapeutic approach, at least two controlled trials of TPE for acute vascular rejection did not find this treatment to be useful (1,2). In contrast, in a more recent controlled trial, Bonomini et al (3) added cyclophosphamide to the standard methylprednisolone pulse therapy and found that the addition of **three to seven plasmapheresis treatments** for antibody-associated rejection resulted in a more rapid decline in anti–human leukocyte antigen (HLA) antibodies, a greater improvement in renal function, and an improved graft survival. It has been pointed out, however, that the episodes of acute rejection described in this report were not typical because the mean interval between transplantation and the onset of rejection was 11 months (4). It should also be noted that none of the available studies using TPE for acute rejection were conducted after the initiation of cyclosporin protocols. Thus, the place for TPE treatment for acute rejection in the age of more modern immunosuppressive regimens remains to be evaluated.

Several recent publications suggested a role for **photopheresis** in the treatment of acute and recurrent renal allograft rejection (5–7), a situation that may mirror the encouraging reports suggesting a role for this technique in the management of heart transplant rejection (8,9).

REFERENCES

1. Kirubakaran MG, Disney APS, Norman J, Pugsley DJ, Mathew TH. A controlled trial of plasmapheresis in the treatment of renal allograft rejection. Transplantation 1981;32:164–165.
2. Allen NH, Dyer P, Geoghegan T, Harris K, Lee HA, Slapak M. Plasma exchange in acute renal allograft rejection. Transplantation 1983;35:425–428.
3. Bonomini V, Vangelista A, Frasca GM, Di Felice A, Liviano D'Arcangelo G. Effects of plasmapheresis in renal transplant rejection: a controlled study. Trans Am Soc Artif Intern Organs 1985;31:698–701.
4. Madore F, Lazarus JM, Brady HR. Therapeutic plasma exchange in renal diseases. J Am Soc Nephrol 1996;7:367-386.
5. Sunder-Plassman G, Druml W, Steininger R, Honigsmann H, Knobler R. Renal allograft rejection controlled by photopheresis. Lancet 1995;346:506.
6. Wolfe JT, Tomaszewski JE, Grossman RA, Gottlieb SL, Naji A, Brayman KL, Kobrin SM, Rook AH. Reversal of acute renal allograft rejection by extracorporeal photopheresis: a case presentation and review of the literature. J Clin Apheresis 1996; 11:36–41.
7. Dall'Amico R, Murer L, Montini G, Andreetta B, Zanon GF, Zacchello G, Zacchello F. Successful treatment of recurrent rejection in renal transplant patients with photopheresis. J Am Soc Nephrol 1998;9:121–127.
8. Dall'Amico R, Livi U, Milano A, Montini G, Andreetta B, Murer L, Zacchello G, Thiene G, Gasarotto D, Zacchello F. Extracor-

poreal photochemotherapy as adjuvant treatment of heart transplant recipients with recurrent rejection. Transplantation 1995; 60:45–49.

9. Costanzo-Nordin MR, Hubbell EA, O'Sullivan EJ, Johnson MR, Mullen GM, Heroux AL, Kao WG, McManus BM, Pifarre R, Robinson JA. Successful treatment of heart transplant rejection with photopheresis. Transplantation 1992;53:808–815.

THE TRANSPLANT CANDIDATE WITH CYTOTOXIC ANTIBODIES

High levels of preformed cytotoxic antibodies against donor ABO, HLA class I, and perhaps other antigens preclude successful renal transplantation because of the risk of hyperacute rejection. Despite the theoretical risk of de novo resynthesis after transplantation, several investigators attempted to manage this problem by the use of protein A columns for the immunoadsorption of plasma reactive antibodies (PRA). Charpentier et al (1) prescribed an average of six immunoadsorbant treatments to lower PRA levels, but results were hampered by a high de novo rate of resynthesis. Nonetheless, with the concomitant administration of cyclophosphamide and prednisolone, 7 of 12 patients were transplantable with a graft survival of 86%. Hakim et al (2) used a similar approach with a mean of eight plasma volumes processed by immunoadsorption, yielding a 40% decline in PRA, but anti-HLA antibodies returned toward pretreatment levels within 4 weeks. More recently, Ross et al (3) reported that four of five hypersensitized patients undergoing this procedure had successful transplants with stable serum creatinines for up to 34 months.

It should be noted that these treatments were performed with a device allowing for the continued regeneration of the protein A columns resulting in a substantial lowering of PRA levels. This device is not currently available in the United States and should not be confused with the Prosorba protein A column, which has a very limited immunoadsorbant capability (see Chap. 3, Selective Removal Techniques: Immunoadsorption). Of note is that the regenerating device used in the above-referenced treatments is designed for the specific adsorption of three of four classes of IgG and will not substantially bind with IgG3, IgA, or IgM. It is not unreasonable to believe that standard plasma exchange, performed with a scheduling of six daily one plasma volume exchanges, would be equally successful in lowering PRA levels with the added potential benefit of removing IgG3, IgA, and IgM. Unfortunately, this type of aggressive plasma exchange scheduling will also entail a depletion coagulopathy that may require a partial replacement with FFP.

Despite the potential usefulness of this approach, the limited amount of available data would lead one to conclude that this aggressive and unconfirmed protocol should not be attempted outside of a well-designed experimental study.

REFERENCES

1. Charpentier BM, Hiesse C, Kriaa F, Rousseau P, Farahmand H, Bismuth A, Fries D. How to deal with the hyperimmunized potential recipients. Kidney Int 1992;42(suppl 38):S176–181.
2. Hakim RM, Milford E, Himmelfarb J, Wingard R, Lazarus J, Watt RM. Extracorporeal removal of anti-HLA antibodies in transplant candidates. Am J Kidney Dis 1990;16:423–431.
3. Ross CN, Gaskin G, Gregor-Macgregor S, Patel AA, Davey NJ, Lechler RI, Williams G, Rees AJ, Pusey CD. Renal transplantation following immunoadsorption in highly sensitized recipients. Transplantation 1993;55:785–789.

Indications for Therapeutic Plasma Exchange in the Intensive Care Unit

13

Fulminant Systemic Meningococcemia   198
TPE for Septic Syndromes Other Than Meningococcemia   201
Burn Shock   205

This chapter reviews the currently available data regarding the use of therapeutic plasma exchange (TPE) as a means of removing endotoxin or other large-molecular-weight substances that are considered to be initiating factors in the cascade of the "septic syndrome" (Table 13-1). The removal of endotoxin represents a promising role for extracorporeal blood purification. In essence, the body has only limited means for clearing these large-molecular-weight toxins that can include fragments of several hundred thousand daltons or more. Under conditions of sepsis, the reticuloendothelial system becomes overloaded and these toxic fragments are trapped in the circulation, stimulating a host of inflammatory processes by way of cytokines, eicosanoids, and nitric oxide. Both standard TPE and selective endotoxin removal by filters impregnated with polymyxin B can successfully remove circulating endotoxins. It should be noted that circulating cytokines may be found in the removed plasma during TPE, but their relatively large volume of distributions and their very short half-lives render TPE a very inefficient means for reducing their serum concentrations. In those

197

Table 13-1.   Indications for TPE in the Intensive Care Unit

	Reference and Year		
	1 1986	2 1993	3 1994
		Rating	
Indications for TPE in the ICU			
Fulminant systemic meningococcemia	nl	nl	nl
Endotoxemia	nl	nl	nl
Burn shock	III	nl	nl

Rating: I, standard therapy, acceptable but not mandatory; II, available evidence tends to favor efficacy: conventional therapy usually tried first; III, inadequately tested at this time; IV, no demonstrated value in controlled trials. nl, not listed; ICU, intensive care unit.

REFERENCES: 1. American Medical Association Council on Scientific Affairs. Current status of therapeutic plasmapheresis. JAMA 1985;253:819–825.
2. Strauss RG, Ciavarella D, Gilcher RO, Kasprisin DO, Kiprov DD, Klein HG, McLeod BC. An overview of current management. J Clin Apheresis 1993;8:189–194.
3. Leitman SF, Ciavarella D, McLeod B, Owen H, Price T, Sniecinski I. Guidelines for therapeutic hemapheresis. Bethesda, MD: American Association of Blood Banks, revised 1994.

few cases in which there has been a documented decrease in serum cytokine levels after TPE, one can assume that the treatment resulted in the removal of a cytokine-inducing substance, such as endotoxin, and that the reduced cytokine levels are a result of a decline in production and not as a result of substantial net removal.

FULMINANT SYSTEMIC MENINGOCOCCEMIA

Fulminant meningococcemia is a syndrome distinct from meningo-coccal meningitis. When severe, it is associated with hypotension, fever, an explosive appearance of disseminated petechiae (in less than 12 hours), relative leukopenia ($<15,000/mm^3$), and thrombo-cytopenia ($<100,000/mm^3$). The Niklasson score, accounting for the above-noted symptoms, predicts a mortality of greater than 70% if three to four of these signs are present (1). Rationale for plasma exchange in the treatment of fulminant meningococcemia is the removal of large-molecular-weight endotoxins. Aside from being implicated as the initiator of a myriad of inflammatory mediators, such as various cytokines and nitric oxide (2), endotoxin is also considered to be the inciting factor in the activation of monocyte-

Table 13-2.   TPE for Fulminant Meningococcemia

Authors	No. of Patients	No. of Survivors	Percent Survivors	Treatment*
Scharfman et al, 1979	1	1	100	PE
Bjorvatn et al, 1984	4	4	100	PE + LP, BE
Brandtzaeg et al, 1985	6	5	83	PE + LP, BE
Brandtzaeg et al, 1989	5	4	80	PE + LP?, BE
Drapkin et al, 1989	1	1	100	PE
Westriendorp et al, 1990	7	5	71	PE + LP, BE
McClelland et al, 1990	1	1	100	PE
van Deuren et al, 1992	15	12	80	PE, BE
Totals	40	33	83	

*PE, plasma exchange: replacement with FFP; LP, leukapheresis; BE, whole blood exchange: in children <30 kg.

derived tissue thromboplastin (3), believed to be a cause of the disseminated intravascular coagulation, which is often the hallmark of this disease. Thus, the removal of endotoxin and monocytes from the circulation has been tried as a means of improving survival.

Since 1979, there have been several anecdotal cases and uncontrolled series reporting the successful use of plasma exchange, with or without leukapheresis, for 33 of 40 patients such treated (Table 13-2) (4–10). The largest series involved 15 cases with a resulting overall survival of 80%, which was substantially improved over the results obtained in 15 consecutive patients previously treated without TPE (10). Furthermore, based on the Niklasson prognostic score, those patients treated with TPE had a predicted mortality of 62% but an actual mortality of only 20%.

Although there are no randomized controlled trials demonstrating the benefits of TPE for fulminant meningococcemia, it should be considered that this is often a desperate illness affecting previously healthy children and young adults in which particularly high levels of endotoxin and inflammatory mediators correlate with an unfavorable outcome (11). Furthermore, the weight of the available evidence is invariably in favor of this approach. **The successful TPE prescription used in the largest series was 30 to 40 mL/kg of plasma exchanged with fresh frozen plasma (FFP) performed as soon as possible after admission and repeated 12 hours later** (10). If the patient's condition remains critical, **further treatments are performed at 24 and 48**

hours. In children weighing less than 25 kg, whole blood exchange was performed with 50 to 60 mL of whole blood per kilogram, following the same schedule. Delay of greater than 40 hours in initiating TPE was associated with a negative outcome.

REFERENCES

1. Niklasson PM, Lundbergh P, Strandell T. Prognostic factors in meningococcal disease. Scand J Infect Dis 1971;3:17–25.
2. Parrillo JE. Pathogenic mechanisms of septic shock. N Engl J Med 1993;328:1471–1477.
3. Osterud B. Meningococcal septicemia: the use of plasmapheresis or blood exchange and how to detect severe endotoxin induced white cell activation. Scand J Clin Lab Invest 1985;45(suppl 178):47–51.
4. Bjorvatn B, Bjertnaes L, Fadnes HO, Flaegstad T, Gutteberg TJ, Kristiansen BE, Pape J, Rekig OP, Osterud B, Aanderud L. Meningococcal septicaemia treated with combined plasmapheresis and leucapheresis or with blood exchange. Br Med J 1984;288:439–441.
5. Brandtzaeg P, Sirnes K, Folsland B, Godal HC, Kierulf P, Bruun JN, Dobloug J. Plasmapheresis in the treatment of severe meningococcal or pneumococcal septicaemia with DIC and fibrinolysis: preliminary data on eight patients. Scand J Clin Lab Invest 1985;45(suppl 178):53–55.
6. Brandtzaeg P, Kierulf P, Gaustad P, Skulberg A, Bruun JN, Halvorsen S, Sorensen E. Plasma endotoxin as a predictor of multiple organ failure and death in systemic meningococcal disease. J Infect Dis 1989;159:195–204.
7. Westindorp RGJ, Brandt A, Thompson J, Dik H, Meinders AE. Experiences with plasma and leucapheresis in meningococcal septicaemia. Int Care Med 1990;16(suppl 1):S102. Abstract.
8. McClelland P, Williams PS, Yaqoob M, Mostafa SM, Bone JM. Multiple organ failure: a role for plasma exchange? Int Care Med 1990;16:100–103.
9. Drapkin MS, Wisch JS, Gelfand JA, Cannon JG, Dinarello CA. Plasmapheresis for fulminant meningococcemia. Pediatr Infect Dis J 1989;8:399–400.
10. van Deuren M, Santman FW, van Dalen R, Sauerwein RW, Span LFR, van der Meer JWM. Plasma and whole blood exchange in meningococcal sepsis. Clin Infect Dis 1992; 15:424–430.

11. Blood exchange and plasmapheresis in sepsis and septic shock. Clin Infect Dis 1992;15:431–433. Editorial.

TPE FOR SEPTIC SYNDROMES OTHER THAN MENINGOCOCCEMIA

Other septic syndromes with assumed endotoxemia may also benefit from TPE (1). A review of English language publications revealed a dozen reports of anecdotal cases and small uncontrolled series involving 82 patients with an overall survival of 73% (Table 13-3) (2–13). The best documented of these reports found that exchange blood transfusion (a common means of performing TPE in neonates) that was successful in removing detectable endotoxin was associated with survival in all of six cases, whereas in the two cases in which treatments were unsuccessful in removing detectable endotoxin, the patients died (4). In contrast, in the least successful of these reports, in which all four patients treated with TPE died, postmortem evaluation determined the existence of persistent foci of infection (8). Clearly, TPE cannot be a sole requirement for survival if the nidus of infection persists; rather, TPE should be considered as a means of assisting in the removal of large-molecular-weight endotoxins but only as an adjunct to successful irradication of the active infection by the appropriate antibiotics or the eventual surgical drainage. Another issue to consider is that of adequate prescription. Clearly, each individual case has a unique rate of endotoxin production and residual endogenous endotoxin clearance. Thus, it is almost impossible to arrive at a generalized recommendation regarding an adequate TPE prescription for endotoxin removal, a question that is all the more evident when study protocols do not result in clinical benefit (14). Nonetheless, in the most successful series, **TPE prescription for endotoxic shock has been reported to range from 2 to 10 TPE procedures, often with FFP as replacement fluid (5,11).** The replaced FFP may have the additional benefit of allowing massive infusion of clotting factors to help reverse an associated disseminated intravascular coagulation.

An alternative to standard plasma exchange is the possibility of endotoxin adsorption, as is accomplished by filters impregnated with polymyxin B, an antibiotic that has the particular propensity to bind endotoxin fragments (see Chap. 3) (15). In early clinical trials, Kodama et al (16) were able to demonstrate a concomitant improvement in systemic hemodynamics as endotoxin levels were

Table 13-3. Blood or Plasma Exchange for Patients with Sepsis/Septic Shock (Excluding Meningococcemia)

Authors/Cultures	No. of Patients	No. of Survivors	Percent Survivors	Treatment
Vain et al, 1980 *Escherichia coli*, group A&B Strep *Haemophilus influenzae*, *Staphylococcus aureus*	10	7	70	BE (infants)
Landini et al, 1981 Leptospirosis	6	6	100	PE
Togari et al, 1983 Serratia, B Strep, Staph Endotoxemia in 8 patients	10	7	70	BE (infants)
Brandtzaeg et al, 1985 *Streptococcus pneumoniae*	2	1	50	PE + LP
Aoki et al, 1987 *E. coli*, Klebsiella, *Pseudomonas aeruginosa*	2	2	100	PE
Graf et al, 1987 Pneumococcus, *Citrobacter freundii*	2	2	100	PE
Hauser et al, 1987 Intraabdominal infections: gram-negative, Candida	4	0	0	PE
Stegmayer and Wirell, 1987 Bacteroides, Clostridia, *Staphylococcus aureus*	4	4	100	PE
Asanuma et al, 1989 Variety of infections	19	13	68	BE (infants)
Stegmayer et al, 1990 Staphylococcus *Escherichia coli*, Clostridia, etc.	15	11	73	PE
McClelland et al, 1990 Candidiasis	1	0	0	PE
Stegmayer et al, 1992 Group A Streptococcus	7	7	100	PE
Totals	82	60	73	

BE, whole blood exchange; PE, plasma exchange with FFP; LP, leukapheresis.

lowered. A more recent report details the results in 16 patients with sepsis-associated multiple organ failure who were treated with 2 hours of polymyxin B hemoperfusion (17). Endotoxin levels decreased from 76 to 21 pg/mL and the pretreatment hyperdynamic cardiac index returned to normal levels. Those patients with pretreatment systolic blood pressures less than 100 mm Hg had substantial increases in blood pressure, whereas fever was reduced for up to 24 hours. Of the 16 patients who underwent the treatment, 9 were alive 2 weeks after and 7 patients were discharged from the hospital, suggesting an improved survival over that which was expected from their pretreatment severity scores.

REFERENCES

1. Stegmayr BG. Plasmapheresis in severe sepsis or septic shock. Blood Purif 1996;14:94–101.
2. Vain NE, Maziumian JR, Swarner W, Cha CC. Role of exchange transfusion in the treatment of severe septicemia. Pediatrics 1980;66:693–697.
3. Landini S, Coli U, Lucatello S, Bassato G. Plasma exchange in severe leptospirosis. Lancet 1981;2:1119–1120.
4. Togari H, Mikawa M, Twanaga T, Matsumoto N, Kawase A, Hagisawa M, Ogino T, Goto R, Watanabe I, Kito H, Ogawa Y, Wada Y. Endotoxin clearance by exchange blood transfusion in septic shock neonates. Acta Paediatr Scand 1983;72:87–91.
5. Brandtzaeg P, Sirnes K, Folsland B, Godal HC, Kierulf P, Bruun JN, Dobloug J. Plasmapheresis in the treatment of severe meningococcal or pneumococcal septicaemia with DIC and fibrinolysis: preliminary data on eight patients. Scand J Clin Lab Invest 1985;45(suppl 178):53–55.
6. Aoki Y, Yukawa H, Katsumi M, Uchita K, Abe T. Successful treatment of endotoxemia by plasma exchange. In: Oda T, Shiokawa Y, Inoue N, eds. Proceedings of the First International Congress of the World Apheresis Association: therapeutic plasmapheresis. Cleveland: ISAO Press, 1987:426–435.
7. Graf N, Bambauer R, Limbach HG, Sitzmann FC, Keuth U. Indications, application and appraisal of therapeutic plasma exchange in children. In: Bambauer R, Malchesky PS, Falkenhagen D, eds. Therapeutic plasma exchange and selective plasma separation. Stuttgart, Schattauer, 1987:267–273.

8. Hauser W, Christmann FJ, Klein T, Traut G. Therapeutic plasma exchange in septic shock. In: Bambauer R, Malchesky PS, Falkenhagen D, eds. Therapeutic plasma exchange and selective plasma separation. Stuttgart, Schattauer, 1987:287–293.

9. Stegmayr B, Wirell M. Reversal of advanced disseminated intravascular coagulation with uremia by plasma exchange. In: Bambauer R, Malchesky PS, Falkenhagen D, eds. Therapeutic plasma exchange and selective plasma separation. Stuttgart, Schattauer, 1987:133–136.

10. Asanuma Y, Takahashi T, Koyama K, Kato T, Omokawa S, Sueoka A, Tanaka J. Exchange blood transfusion and on-line plasma exchange for sepsis in infants. Am Soc Artif Intern Organs Trans 1989;35:343–345.

11. Stegmayr B, Berseus O, Bjorsell-Ostling E, Wirell M. Plasma exchange in patients with severe consumption coagulopathy and acute renal failure. Transfus Sci 1990;11:271–277.

12. McClelland P, Williams PS, Yaqoob M, Mostafa SM, Bone JM. Multiple organ failure—a role for plasma exchange? Int Care Med 1990;16:100–103.

13. Stegmayr B, Bjorch S, Holm S, Nisell J, Rydvall A, Settergren B. Septic shock induced by group A streptococcal infection: clinical and therapeutic aspects. Scand J Infect Dis 1992; 24:589–597.

14. Natanson C, Hoffman WD, Danner RL, Koev LL, Banks SM, Walker LD, Heyman P, Parrillo JE. A controlled trial of plasmapheresis fails to improve outcome in an antibiotic treated canine model of human septic shock. Transfusion 1993;33: 243–248.

15. Hanasawa K, Aoki H, Yoshioka T, Matsuda K, Tani T, Kodama M. Novel mechanical assistance in the treatment of endotoxic and septicemic shock. Am Soc Artif Intern Organs Trans 1989;35:341–343.

16. Kodama M, Aoki H, Tani T, Hanasawa K. Hemoperfusion using a polymyxin B immobilized fiber column for the removal of endotoxin. In: Levin J, Alving CR, Munford RS, Stutz PL, eds. Bacterial endotoxin: recognition and effector mechanisms. Amsterdam: Elsevier Science Publishers B.V., 1993:389–398.

17. Aoki H, Kodama M, Tani T, Hanasawa K. Treatment of sepsis by extracorporeal elimination of endotoxin using polymyxin B-immobilized fiber. Am J Surg 1994;167:412–417.

BURN SHOCK

The vascular collapse associated with burn shock has been attributed to circulating inflammatory mediators. As such, TPE has been evaluated as a potential means for assisting in the resuscitation of these patients. An early retrospective review demonstrated that TPE could improve the therapeutic response to standard resuscitation procedures, with decreased lactic acidosis and increased urine output (1). The same group followed with a controlled study of 22 patients randomized to receive standard resuscitation procedures with or without TPE (2). The group receiving **TPE was given a single 1 to 1.5 times plasma volume exchange with FFP, performed as soon as possible after admission**. Resuscitation was completed earlier (20 versus 30 hours) and adequate urine output was achieved sooner in the group receiving TPE.

REFERENCES

1. Warden GD, Stratta RJ, Saffle JR, Kravitz M, Ninnemann JL. Plasma exchange therapy in patients failing to resuscitate from burn shock. J Trauma 1983;23:945–951.
2. Kravitz M, Warden GD, Sullivan JJ, Saffle JR. A randomized trial of plasma exchange in the treatment of burn shock. J Burn Care Rehabil 1989;10:17–26.

Therapeutic Plasma Exchange in Patients with Human Immunodeficiency Virus

14

General Comments   207
Risk of Accidental HIV Transmission to Patients and Staff   208
Immune Thrombocytopenic Purpura   209
Thrombotic Thrombocytopenic Purpura/Hemolytic Uremic Syndrome   209
Peripheral Neuropathy   210

Despite early attempts to use plasma exchange as an immunomodulating treatment for patients with human immunodeficiency virus (HIV) infection (1), this treatment is most commonly reserved as a means of treating HIV-related syndromes for which therapeutic plasma exchange (TPE) has been shown to be effective in the non–HIV-infected population. Included in this list of syndromes are idiopathic thrombocytopenic purpura, thrombotic thrombocytopenic purpura/hemolytic uremic syndrome (TTP/HUS), demyelinating peripheral neuropathy, and hyperviscosity syndrome. TPE for patients with HIV infection has also been used in syndromes for which its efficacy has been less well established in the non–HIV-infected population such as autoimmune neutropenia and immune complex–mediated disorders (2).

Indications for TPE in patients with HIV are listed and rated in Table 14-1. An abbreviated review of the evidence for TPE efficacy in these HIV-related disorders is given in this chapter, but the reader is strongly encouraged to refer to the more extensive

Table 14-1. Indications for TPE in Patients with HIV

	Reference and Year		
	1 1986	2 1993	3 1994
	Rating		
HIV	III	nl	nl
Immune thrombocytopenic purpura	nl	II	nl
Thrombotic thrombocytopenic purpura	nl	I	nl
Peripheral neuropathy	nl	I	nl

Rating: I, standard therapy, acceptable but not mandatory; II, available evidence tends to favor efficacy: conventional therapy usually tried first; III, inadequately tested at this time; IV, no demonstrated value in controlled trials. nl, not listed.
REFERENCES: 1. American Medical Association Council on Scientific Affairs. Current status of therapeutic plasmapheresis. JAMA 1985;253:819–825.
2. Strauss RG, Ciavarella D, Gilcher RO, Kasprisin DO, Kiprov DD, Klein HG, McLeod BC. An overview of current management. J Clin Apheresis 1993;8:189–194.
3. Leitman SF, Ciavarella D, McLeod B, Owen H, Price T, Sniecinski I. Guidelines for therapeutic hemapheresis. Bethesda, MD: American Association of Blood Banks, revised 1994.

discussion presented for each of these syndromes in the appropriate sections elsewhere in this volume.

REFERENCES

1. Tomar RH, Kloster BE, Lamberson HV. Plasmapheresis increases T4 lymphocytes in a patient with AIDS. Am J Clin Pathol 1984;81:518–552.
2. Kiprov DD, Strauss RG, Ciavarella D, Gilcher RO, Kasprisin DO, Klein HG, McLeod BC. Management of autoimmune disorders. J Clin Apheresis 1993;8:195–210.

GENERAL COMMENTS

Most immune-based disorders treated with TPE require an immunosuppressive regimen involving steroids and/or cytotoxic agents for maintenance of remission. The immunodepression associated with HIV infection renders this strategy problematic and may, in fact, lend support to the use of TPE, which may help to limit the use of these agents. Nonetheless, each clinical situation must be viewed as unique and the physician must weigh risks and benefits to each therapeutic manipulation. In those situations in which 5% albumin would normally be the replacement fluid of choice, the resulting immunoglobulin depletion has led some authors to advocate the use of post–TPE infusions of intravenous immunoglobulin (IVIG) to restore the lost immunity. Kiprov et al (1) recommended the immediate post-treatment infusion of 250 mg/kg of IVIG in those patients requiring chronic repetitive treatments, such as a once weekly exchange for those with polyneuropathy who have originally responded to the more extensive initial treatment.

RISK OF ACCIDENTAL HIV TRANSMISSION TO PATIENTS AND STAFF

HIV transmission to health professionals involved with the TPE treatments is an obvious concern. Implementation of universal precautions and careful attention to accident-free procedures virtually eliminates any possibility of transmission. Recommended practices include the use of gloves, the covering of open skin lesions, the use of protective eye wear, and the use of appropriate disposal containers (2,3).

Although the thrust of this chapter involves the use of TPE as a treatment for HIV-related syndromes, it is appropriate to consider the risks of HIV transmission to non–HIV-infected patients receiving TPE for unrelated disorders. In this regard, there has been a documented case of HIV infection in a patient treated for Guillain-Barré syndrome for whom transmission occurred as a result of the TPE treatment (4). Although this report dates from a period in which screening for HIV-infected plasma was less well established, this type of occurrence lends credence to the use of replacement fluids in which viral transmission of any type is unlikely or impossible (heat-treated albumin, hetastarch, etc.). Aside from the minimal risks currently encountered as a result of HIV-infected plasma (1/680,000 units [5–7]), residual contamination of the apheresis equipment after treatment of an HIV-infected patient should be considered. In this regard, the best policy is the use of disposable products for all equipment in direct contact with blood, such as tubing, filters, bowls, belts, membranes, needles, and syringes. The machine should be cleaned with a disinfectant, and all blood spills should be decontaminated with bleach. Given these precautions, transmission of HIV to patients or staff is very unlikely, and in a large series involving over 100 TPE-treated patients and their attendant staff, despite concurrent treatment of patients with documented pretreatment HIV infection, no such transmission was documented (8).

IMMUNE THROMBOCYTOPENIC PURPURA

As in patients without HIV, immune thrombocytopenic purpura (ITP) has been successfully treated with plasma adsorption over a staph A column (Prosorba, Cypress Bioscience, San Diego, CA). Mittleman et al (9) treated 29 patients with HIV-associated ITP and achieved a 170 to 450% increase in platelet counts with a duration of between 8 and 12 months. **Treatment prescription involved the removal of 250 mL of plasma and its perfusion over the staph A column. Four to eight treatments were performed on a weekly schedule.** The most common secondary effects occurred with a frequency of between 5 and 29% and included fever, chills, pain, nausea/vomiting, and rash but required minimal or no therapy. Pretreatment with diphenhydramine and acetaminophen may decrease the incidence of these reactions (1). In what was an apparent follow-up review, Snyder et al (10) reported on 37 patients, with a reported response in 18 (49%). Treatment prescription was noted as an average of six treatments over a 3-week period. Aside from the previously noted treatment-related toxicities, a delayed reaction involving urticaria and joint pain was noted in seven patients and treated with antihistamines. A serum sickness-like reaction involving a transient vasculitis of the lower extremities was noted in two patients.

THROMBOTIC THROMBOCYTOPENIC PURPURA/HEMOLYTIC UREMIC SYNDROME

Both TTP and HUS have been noted in HIV-infected patients. In an early report, two patients with what was then described as "[acquired immunodeficiency syndrome] AIDS-related complex" were found to have classic symptoms and laboratory findings of TTP and were successfully treated with aspirin, dipyridamole, prednisone, and TPE (11). **Treatment prescription involved daily exchanges with fresh frozen plasma (FFP) (2000 to 2300 mL) for 2 to 3 weeks.** Thompson et al (12), using a prescription of daily large-volume exchanges with FFP, reported initial treatment success in six of seven patients, but no patient survived more than 2 years after the initial episode. More recently, Badesha and Saklayen (13) described a patient who presented with HUS-related renal failure who was subsequently found to have occult HIV infection. Despite 14 courses of TPE, there was no improvement, and treatment was subsequently withdrawn. In a review of the literature, these authors were able to document 43 cases of TTP/HUS in HIV-infected patients. Despite the failure of TPE in their report, the authors concluded that TPE was still considered a successful treatment option in many HIV patients. Gadallah et al (14) combined the TTP/HUS complex into a single entity labeled thrombotic microangiopathy (TMA) and reviewed the records of 214 patients with HIV infection and found that 15 patients (7%) had evidence of TMA at the time of their death. They concluded that TMA is common in AIDS patients and that HIV-associated TMA has a good prognosis similar to that of idiopathic TMA, whereas AIDS-associated TMA has a grave prognosis. In the current context of protease inhibitors and changing definitions of HIV infection, such distinctions may no longer be relevant.

PERIPHERAL NEUROPATHY

A variety of forms of peripheral neuropathy may be associated with HIV infection and its treatment (15). Distal symmetric polyneuropathy may be produced by neurotoxic drugs (vincristine, isoniazid [INH], 2'3'-dideoxyinosine [ddI] or dideoxycytidine [ddC]), vitamin B_{12} deficiency, or as a result of autoimmune mechanisms such as with Guillain-Barré syndrome or chronic inflammatory demyelinating polyneuropathy. Although cytomegalovirus infection is most commonly associated with a mononeuropathy multiplex, a demyelinating form of polyneuropathy has also been described (16). Because only the autoimmune-based neuropathies are likely to respond to TPE, it is essential that a proper neurologic evaluation is performed before the initiation of any therapeutic maneuvers. In fact, evidence for autoimmunity may not be sufficient to ensure response to TPE. Kiprov et al (17) evaluated 30 HIV-positive patients with peripheral neuropathies and autoimmunity as evident by the presence of antibodies against peripheral nerve tissue. Six of these patients underwent a series of TPE, but clinical improvement was only noted in the four patients in whom there was evidence of a demyelinating type of neuropathy (slowed nerve conduction studies). In this series, **successful TPE prescription was one plasma volume exchange performed every other day for 3**

weeks. Replacement fluid was 5% albumin. In some, additional maintenance treatments were performed once every 2 weeks for 2 months. In two patients, a repeat series was performed several months later because of relapse. Similar success has been described by other authors in small series or case reports (18–20).

REFERENCES

1. Kiprov DD, Strauss RG, Ciavarella D, Gilcher RO, Kasprisin DO, Klein HG, McLeod BC. Management of autoimmune disorders. J Clin Apheresis 1993;8:195–210.
2. Kiprov DD, Lippert R, Miller RG, Sandstrom E, Jones FR, Cohen RJ, Abrams D, Busch DF. The use of plasmapheresis, lymphocytapheresis, and staph protein-A immunoadsorption as an immunomodulatory therapy in patients with AIDS and AIDS-related conditions. J Clin Apheresis 1986;3:133–139.
3. Kiprov DD, Simpson DM, Pfaeffl W, Romanick-Schmiedl S, Abrams D, Miller RG. AIDS and apheresis procedures—therapeutic and safety considerations. Blood Purif 1987;5:51–56.
4. Boucher CA, de Gans J, van Oers R, Danner S, Goudsmit J. Transmission of HIV and AIDS by plasmapheresis for Guillain-Barré syndrome. Clin Neurol Neurosurg 1988;90:235–236.
5. Lackritz EM, Satten GA, Aberle-Grasse J, et al. Estimated risk of transmission of the human immunodeficiency virus by screened blood in the United States. N Engl J Med 1995;333:1721–1725.
6. Schreiber GB, Busch MP, Kleinman SH, Korelitz JJ. The risk of transfusion-transmitted virus infections. The Retrovirus Epidemiology Donor Study. N Engl J Med 1996;334:1685–1690.
7. AuBuchon JP, Birkmeyer JD, Busch MP. Safety of the blood supply in the United States: opportunities and controversies. Ann Intern Med 1997;127:904–909.
8. Kiprov D, Simpson D, Romanick-Schmiedl S, et al. Risk of AIDS-related virus (human immunodeficiency virus) transmission through apheresis procedures. J Clin Apheresis 1987;3:143–146.
9. Mittleman A, Bertram J, Henry DH, Snyder HW Jr, Messerschmidt GL, Ciavarella D, Ainsworth S, Kiprov D,

Arlin Z. Treatment of patients with HIV thrombocytopenia and hemolytic uremic syndrome with protein A (Prosorba column) immunoadsorption. Semin Hematol 1989;26(suppl a):15–18.

10. Snyder H Jr, Bertram JH, Henry DH, Kiprov DD, Benny WB, Mittleman A, Messerschmidt GL, Cochran SK, Perkins W, Balint JP Jr, Jones FR. Use of protein A immunoadsorption as a treatment for thrombocytopenia in HIV-infected homosexual men: a retrospective evaluation of 37 cases. AIDS 1991;5:1257–1260.

11. Nair JM, Bellevue R, Bertoni M, Dosik H. Thrombotic thrombocytopenic purpura in patients with the acquired immunodeficiency syndrome (AIDS)-related complex. A report of two cases. Ann Intern Med 1988;109:209–212.

12. Thompson CE, Damon LE, Ries CA, Linker CA. Thrombotic microangiopathies in the 1980's: clinical features, response to treatment and the impact of the human immunodeficiency virus epidemic. Blood 1992;80:1890–1895.

13. Badesha PS, Saklayen MG. Hemolytic uremic syndrome as a presenting form of HIV infection. Nephron 1996;72:472–475.

14. Gadallah MF, el-Shahawy MA, Campese VM, Todd JR, King JW. Disparate prognosis of thrombotic microangiopathy in HIV-infected patients with and without AIDS. Am J Nephrol 1996;16:446–450.

15. Simpson DM, Olney RK. Peripheral neuropathies associated with human immunodeficiency virus infection. Neurol Clin 1992;10:685–711.

16. Morgello S, Simpson DM. Multifocal cytomegalovirus demyelinative polyneuropathy associated with AIDS. Muscle Nerve 1994;17:176–182.

17. Kiprov D, Pfaeffl W, Parry G, Lippert R, Lang W, Miller R. Antibody-mediated peripheral neuropathies associated with ARC and AIDS: successful treatment with plasmapheresis. J Clin Apheresis 1988;4:3–7.

18. Wuest D, Goldfinger D. Plasmapheresis in the treatment of acute relapsing inflammatory demyelinating polyradiculoneuropathy associated with human immunodeficiency virus infection: a case report. J Clin Apheresis 1988;4:149–151.

19. Salim YS, Faber V, Skinhoj P, Lerche B, Soeberg B, Mikkelsen S, Klinken L, Trojaborg W, Jakobsen J, Kamieniecka Z, et al. Plasmapheresis in the treatment of peripheral HIV neuropathy.

Ugeskr Laeger 1989;151:1754–1756. In Dutch, abstract in English.

20. Alpert JN, Loar C, DePriest J, Sermas A, Merritt L. Polyradiculoneuropathy in transfusion-associated AIDS and dorsal root pathology. Tex Med 1989;85:45–48.

Intoxications

15

General Guidelines for the Use of TPE in the Treatment of Intoxications   215
Arsine   217
Carbamazepine   218
Cisplatin   218
Digitoxin Overdose   220
Digoxin-Specific Antibody Fragments   221
Diltiazem   221
Mushrooms: *Amanita phalloides* and *Amanita verna*   222
Mushrooms: Cortinarius   224
Mushrooms: *Paxillus involutus*   225
Paraquat Poisoning   225
Parathion Poisoning   226
Phenylbutazone   227
Phenytoin   227
Quinine   228
Sodium Chlorate Intoxication   229
Theophylline   229
Thyroxine   230
Tricyclic Antidepressants   230
Vincristine   232
Miscellaneous Intoxications   232

In general, therapeutic plasma exchange (TPE) is most useful for the removal of toxins that have a high percentage of protein binding (>90%) and a relatively modest volume of distribution (<0.6 L/kg). Those intoxications that have been treated by TPE are listed below in Table 15-1. In some cases, the drug's volume of distribution was so large that TPE removal was insignificant.

Table 15-1. TPE for Intoxications

	Reference and Year		
	1 1986	2 1993	3 1994
		Rating	
Intoxications	I	II	II
Arsine			
Carbamazepine (TPE is not useful)			
Cisplatin			
Digitoxin			
Digoxin			
Diltiazem			
Mushroom poisoning			
Amanita phalloides		II	
Cortinarius orellanus			
Paxillus involutus			
Paraquat		II	
Parathion		II	
Phenylbutazone			
Phenytoin			
Quinine (TPE is not useful)			
Sodium chlorate		II	
Theophylline			
Thyroxine			
Tricyclic antidepressant (TPE is not useful)			
Vincristine			
Miscellaneous			

Rating: I, standard therapy, acceptable but not mandatory; II, available evidence tends to favor efficacy: conventional therapy usually tried first; III, inadequately tested at this time; IV, no demonstrated value in controlled trials.

REFERENCES: 1. American Medical Association Council on Scientific Affairs. Current status of therapeutic plasmapheresis. JAMA 1985;253:819–825.
2. Strauss RG, Ciavarella D, Gilcher RO, Kasprisin DO, Kiprov DD, Klein HG, McLeod BC. An overview of current management. J Clin Apheresis 1993;8:189–194.
3. Leitman SF, Ciavarella D, McLeod B, Owen H, Price T, Sniecinski I. Guidelines for therapeutic hemapheresis. Bethesda, MD: American Association of Blood Banks, revised 1994.

GENERAL GUIDELINES FOR THE USE OF TPE IN THE TREATMENT OF INTOXICATIONS

As a general rule, TPE is only an efficient blood purification treatment for those poisons or drugs that have a high percentage of protein binding and a relatively modest volume of distribution (<0.6 L/kg) (1–3). Assuming the simplest pharmacokinetics, the volume of plasma exchanged would have to equal 0.7 times the volume of distribution of the drug or poison to remove 50% of the body's total burden (see Chap. 2). For example, a TPE treatment would have to exchange 7 liters of plasma to remove 50% of a drug whose volume of distribution is a modest 0.15 L/kg (~10 liters in a 70-kg patient). Given this basic tenet, even a drug that is more than 90% protein bound would be minimally removed if its volume of distribution was at least 0.6 L/kg ($\geq$42 liters in a 70-kg patient). It is therefore not surprising that TPE has not become a widely used means of blood purification for the treatment of drug intoxications, despite the fact that many drugs are highly protein bound (see Table 5-2).

Gadow and Sprenger (4) reviewed the blood purification capabilities of the available techniques (hemodialysis, hemoperfusion, and TPE) and concluded that TPE is best suited for those situations in which a lethal or highly toxic dose of a poison or drug has been ingested, endogenous clearance is less than 500 mL/min, protein binding is greater than 90%, and the volume of distribution is less than 0.6 L/kg. References 5 through 10 provide general reviews of the use of TPE for the treatment of intoxications. Although limited in its discussion of TPE, reference 11 provides a comprehensive review of the basic pharmacokinetics that govern the treatment of intoxications.

REFERENCES

1. Kaplan AA, Halley SE. Plasma exchange with a rotating filter. Kidney Int 1990;38:160–166.
2. Sketris IS, Parker WA, Jones JV. Effect of plasma exchange on drug removal. In: Valbonesi M, Pineda AA, Biggs JC, eds. Therapeutic hemapheresis. Milano: Wichtig Editore, 1986:15–20.
3. Jones JV. The effect of plasmapheresis on therapeutic drugs. Dial Transplant 1985;14:225–226.
4. Gadow KA, Sprenger KB. Successful plasmapheresis in severe diltiazem poisoning. Dtsch Med Wochenschr 1995;120:1023–1024. In German.
5. Li PK, Lai KN. Active therapeutic approaches to drug intoxication. Adverse Drug React Acute Poison Rev 1988;7:55–73.
6. Jones JS, Dougherty J. Current status of plasmapheresis in toxicology. Ann Emerg Med 1986;15:474–482.

7. Lembeck F, Beubler E, Lepuschutz HF, Stolze A. Plasmapheresis in the elimination of toxic substances with marked plasma protein-binding properties. Wien Klin Wochenschr 1977;89: 257–260. In German.
8. Larsen LS, Sterrett JR, Whitehead B, Marcus SM. Adjunctive therapy of phenytoin overdose—a case report using plasmaphoresis. J Toxicol Clin Toxicol 1986;24:37–49.
9. Wenz B, Barland P. Therapeutic intensive plasmapheresis. Semin Hematol 1981;18:147–162.
10. Peterson RG, Peterson LN. Cleansing the blood. Hemodialysis, peritoneal dialysis, exchange transfusion, charcoal hemoperfusion, forced diuresis. Pediatr Clin North Am 1986;33: 675–689.
11. Winchester JF. Poisoning: is the role of the nephrologist diminishing? Am J Kidney Dis 1989;13:171–183.

ARSINE

Arsine results when metals containing arsenic are exposed to acids (1). Renal failure results from a Coombs'-negative hemolytic anemia and the resulting hemoglobinuria. Two cases of arsine poisoning were treated with hemodialysis, dimercaprol British antilewisite (BAL), and exchange transfusion (2). Exchange transfusion was most likely useful as a means of removing free hemoglobin to avoid renal toxicity. Standard TPE would probably provide the same benefit because it is known to be able to remove free hemoglobin and reduce serum levels (3). More recently, occupational arsine poisoning was described in a small family workshop during blackening operations on zinc/aluminum alloy parts (4).

REFERENCES

1. Hall AH, Robertson WO. Arsenic and other heavy metals. In: Haddad LM, Winchester JF, eds. Clinical management of poisoning and drug overdose. 2nd ed. Philadelphia: WB Saunders, 1990:1027–1028.
2. Dllhopolcek P, Hrnciar J, Dalik R., Kolacny J, Find'o P, Szentivanyi M. Acute industrial poisoning with arsine. Vnitr Lek 1982;28:393–398. In Slovak.
3. Larsen LS, Sterrett JR, Whitehead B, Marcus SM. Adjunctive therapy of phenytoin overdose—a case report using plasmaphoresis. J Toxicol Clin Toxicol 1986;24:37–49.

4. Marchiori L, Rozio L, Bressan A, Biasoli S, Cesaro A, Peretti A, Tommasi I, Perbellini L. Occupational arsine poisoning: description of a case. Med Lav 1989;80:330–334. In Italian.

CARBAMAZEPINE

Carbamazepine overdose causes neurotoxicity in the form of coma, convulsions, drowsiness, ataxia, nystagmus, vomiting, and dystonia (1). In 27 patients with moderate coma, the mean serum level of carbamazepine was 112 μmol/L (range, 63 to 176). In 45 patients whose conscious state was mildly depressed or normal, the mean serum level was 73 μmol/L (range, 37 to 128). After review of the available data, Tibballs (1) concluded that patients with serum carbamazepine levels of approximately 100 μmol/L require close observation, whereas those with levels greater than 150 μmol/L may require intensive life support. Carbamazepine has a volume of distribution listed between 0.8 and 1.6 L/kg, or about 56 to 112 liters in a 70-kg patient. Thus, it is not surprising that despite a 75% protein binding, **the available evidence would suggest that TPE is *not* an efficient means for the removal of this drug**. In one reported case, overdose with 5.9 g of carbamazepine was treated with three TPE treatments, resulting in a total removal of only 336 mg of drug (2). Although drug clearance increased by almost 70% during the TPE treatments, there was a 40% rebound after the first treatment and an 18% rebound after the second treatment. The authors also stated that TPE did not seem to have a great impact on the patient's clinical status. In conclusion, they found it difficult to recommend plasmapheresis in the treatment of an acute overdose.

REFERENCES

1. Tibballs J. Acute toxic reaction to carbamazepine: clinical effects and serum concentrations. J Pediatr 1992;121:295–299.
2. Kale PB, Thomson PA, Provenzano R, Higgins MJ. Evaluation of plasmapheresis in the treatment of an acute overdose of carbamazepine. Ann Pharmacother 1993;27:866–870.

CISPLATIN

Cisplatin is a platinum-based combination chemotherapeutic agent that has significantly improved the treatment of certain neoplasms, such as ovarian, germ cell, lung, and head and neck cancer. It is the first-line chemotherapeutic agent in ovarian cancers. Cisplatin is one of the most potent chemotherapeutic agents, but its use is limited because of its serious nephrotoxic effects (1,2). Cisplatin is 90% protein bound and has an estimated volume of distribution of only 0.5 L/kg, suggesting that TPE may be useful in the management of cisplatin overdose. Two such cases have been reported. In one case, a 59-year-old man received a massive cisplatin overdose of 300 mg/m² (3). Toxicities included severe emesis, myelosuppression, renal failure, and mental deterioration with hallucination, dim vision, and hepatic toxicity. Plasmapheresis was effective in lowering the platinum concentration from **2979 to 185 ng/mL** and appeared to be of clinical benefit. Granulocyte macrophage colony-stimulating factor (GM-CSF) was used to ameliorate myelosuppression. The patient's renal function was restored 3 months later and partial response of esophageal cancer was obtained. Another case involved the accidental substitution of cisplatin for carboplatin in which a 68-year-old woman received a massive overdose of cisplatin without intravenous hydration (4). As in the previous case, toxicities included severe emesis, myelosuppression, renal failure, and deafness. Other toxicities were seizures, hallucinations, loss of vision, and hepatic toxicity, which were unusual and may have been caused by the magnitude of the overdose. As late as day 19, there was a continued cellular response from cisplatin. Plasmapheresis was effective in lowering the platinum concentration from greater than **2900 to 200 ng/mL** and appeared to be of clinical benefit. Even after the onset of renal failure, hydration to increase urine volume resulted in increased urinary excretion of platinum. GM-CSF was used to ameliorate myelosuppression. The patient received a transplanted kidney from her monozygotic twin sister and survived with no clinically significant deficit except for deafness.

Measurement of cisplatin concentrations can be made by atomic absorption spectroscopy (3,4) and by xeroderma pigmentosum group E binding factor, a protein that is involved in the recognition step of DNA repair (4).

REFERENCES

1. Ozols RF, Young RC. High dose cisplatin therapy in ovarian cancer. Semin Oncol 1985;12:21–30.
2. Cornelison TL, Reed E. Nephrotoxicity and hydration man-

agement for cisplatin, carboplatin, and ormaplatin. Gynecol Oncol 1993;50:147–158.
3. Jung HK, Lee J, Lee SN. A case of massive cisplatin overdose managed by plasmapheresis. Korean J Intern Med 1995;10:150–154.
4. Chu G, Mantin R, Shen YM, Baskett G, Sussman H. Massive cisplatin overdose by accidental substitution for carboplatin. Toxicity and management. Cancer 1993;72:3707–3714.

DIGITOXIN OVERDOSE

Digitoxin overdose may lead to severe ventricular arrhythmias resistant to antiarrhythmic medication. Despite a 94% protein binding, volume of distribution is estimated at 0.6 L/kg. Although TPE removes only 3% of the body load, this has been reported to be sufficient to alleviate acute cardiac toxicity (1,2). In one report, net digitoxin removal was determined for hemodialysis, hemofiltration, hemoperfusion, and TPE, revealing a substantially greater removal with TPE (3). In another report, **a 3.5-liter exchange with albumin produced a decrease in digitoxin level from 124 to less than 50 nM/L (maximal therapeutic level is 32 nM/L) (4). These same authors described a rebound within 48 hours and recommended a repeat TPE treatment within 36 to 48 hours after the first treatment.** Because there is substantial intraerythrocytic distribution, a whole blood exchange may be more efficient.

REFERENCES

1. Seyffart G. Plasmapheresis in treatment of acute intoxications. Trans Am Soc Artif Intern Organs 1982;28:673–676.
2. Jones JS, Dougherty J. Current status of plasmapheresis in toxicology. Ann Emerg Med 1986;15:474–482.
3. Peters U, Risler T, Grabenese B. Digitoxin elimination by plasma separation. In: Sieberth HG, ed. Plasma exchange: plasmapheresis-plasmaseparation. Stuttgart: FK Schattauer Verlag, 1980:365–368.
4. Arsac PH, Barret L, Chenais F, Debru JL, Faure J. Digitoxin intoxication treated by plasma exchange. In: Sieberth HG, ed. Plasma exchange: plasmapheresis-plasmaseparation. Stuttgart: FK Schattauer Verlag, 1980:369–371.

DIGOXIN-SPECIFIC ANTIBODY FRAGMENTS

Digoxin-specific antibody Fab fragments (Digibind, Glaxo-Wellcome, Research Triangle Park, NC) have been used to treat digoxin intoxication. The fragments have a molecular weight of 50,000 Da, and the digoxin-Fab fragments are normally excreted by glomerular filtration. In cases associated with significant renal failure, excretion of the digoxin-bound fragments is prolonged from a normal duration of 1 hour to as much as 24 hours or more. This prolonged half-life results in a risk of rebound toxicity as digoxin is released from the Fab complex. Under these conditions, it has been suggested that TPE, performed 24 to 48 hours after infusion of the Fab fragments, may prevent this late digoxin toxicity (1). In the case reported, **TPE exchange was 3 liters on the first day and 4.2 liters on the second day**. A substantial decline in the digibind level was achieved after the second treatment and a rebound phenomenon did not occur.

REFERENCE

1. Rabetoy GM, Price CA, Findlay JW, Sailstad JM. Treatment of digoxin intoxication in a renal failure patient with digoxin-specific antibody fragments and plasmapheresis. Am J Nephrol 1990;10:518–521.

DILTIAZEM

Diltiazem is a calcium channel blocker that can cause heart block, bradyarrhythmias, myocardial depression, and hypotension. The drug is 98% protein bound and has an estimated volume of distribution of between 3 and 5 L/kg. This enormous volume of distribution would appear to preclude any appreciable net removal by TPE, but Gutschmidt (1) described a case of diltiazem overdose involving the ingestion of 7.2 g of drug in which TPE lowered levels from 2292 to 798 ng/mL after the first treatment and to 187 ng/mL after the second treatment. Despite the apparent success of these treatments, two subsequent letters provided considerable criticism to the conclusion that TPE provided significant drug removal (2,3). Calculating from the published report, these authors conclude that the net removal of drug during the first treatment was only 6.2 mg, or only 0.09% of the ingested amount

([2292 ng/mL + 798 ng/mL]/2 × 4000 mL [estimated plasma volume] = 6.2 mg). Nonetheless, the possibility remains that the substantial lowering of plasma levels provided by the TPE treatment may have been useful in limiting cardiotoxicity.

REFERENCES

1. Gutschmidt HJ. Successful plasmapheresis in severe diltiazem poisoning. Dtsch Med Wochenschr 1995;120:81–82. In German.
2. Samtleben W. Successful plasmapheresis in severe diltiazem poisoning. Dtsch Med Wochenschr 1995;120:1023. In German.
3. Gadow KA, Sprenger KB. Successful plasmapheresis in severe diltiazem poisoning. Dtsch Med Wochenschr 1995;120:1023–1024. In German.

MUSHROOMS: *AMANITA PHALLOIDES* AND *AMANITA VERNA*

Amanitin is highly hepatotoxic and is tightly bound to serum proteins. Fatalities are common with ingestion of as little as three mushrooms (50 g) (1). An early phase of gastrointestinal upset with abdominal pain, diarrhea, and vomiting occurs between 8 and 12 hours after ingestion. Although these symptoms may respond to conventional therapy, liver function tests reveal increasing levels of transaminases. Eventually, jaundice, circulatory collapse, hemorrhage, and renal failure are seen. Mortality is often 50% or more. Although hemoperfusion over charcoal has been reported to be successful in removing the highly protein-bound amanitin toxin (1), TPE performed with currently available machines may be a more efficient means of removing the toxin. In one report, 17 patients were successfully treated with TPE with a substantial lowering of expected mortality (2). Prescription was with exchanges of 60 mL/kg of body weight, and fresh frozen plasma replacement was recommended if clotting parameters were abnormal. If transaminases did not improve with TPE, a second treatment was performed. Despite the apparent success of this approach, a recent review suggested that the concomitant administration of thioctic acid, an experimental drug with its own reported success, clouds the interpretation of this result (3). In another series, 10 patients were treated with gastric lavage, oral carbo medicinalis, and saline laxans, combined with intravenous dextrose and saline, penicillin, and hydrocortisone (4). TPE was performed between 38 and 46 hours after ingestion. Total volume exchanged was approximately 4% of body weight in the first five patients and 10% in the next five patients. Nine patients survived, suggesting a substantial benefit to this combined approach. In a series involving 87 patients, a significant difference between elevation of serum transaminases and prolongation of prothrombin time was found in patients receiving TPE and competitive inhibition with penicillin or silibinin, as compared with those receiving TPE alone (5). In another report involving 53 patients, forced diuresis was found to be the most useful means of toxin removal, being far more efficient than TPE (6).

Because of the greater popularity of eating wild mushrooms in Europe, there are a multitude of reports of *Amanita phalloides* intoxications in the non-English literature (7–12). There are no simple methods for distinguishing edible mushrooms from poisonous ones (9).

REFERENCES

1. Mushroom poisoning. Lancet 1980;2:351–352. Editorial.
2. Mercuriali R, Sirchia G. Plasma exchange for mushroom poisoning. Transfusion 1977;17:644–646.
3. Kasprisin DO, Strauss RG, Ciavarella D, Gilcher RO, Kiprov DD, Klein HG, McLeod BC. Management of metabolic and miscellaneous disorders. J Clin Apheresis 1993;8:231–241.
4. Ponikvar R, Drinovec J, Kandus A, Varl J, Gucek A, Malovrh M. Plasma exchange in management of severe acute poisoning with amanita phalloides. In: Rock G, ed. Apheresis. New York: Wiley-Liss, 1990:327–329.
5. Gasparovic V, Puljevic D, Radonic R, Gjurasin M, Ivanovic D, De Wollf F, Pisl Z. Mushroom poisoning with a long period of development. Lijec Vjesn 1991;113:16–20. In Serbo-Croatian (Roman).
6. Vesconi S, Langer M, Iapichino G, Costantino D, Busi C, Fiume L. Therapy of cytotoxic mushroom intoxication. Crit Care Med 1985;13:402–406.
7. Russo GE, Giusti S, Maurici M, Bosco M, Vitaliano E, Caramiello MS, Bauco B, De Marco CM, Marigliano V. Plasmapheresis and mushroom poisoning: report of a case of Amanita phalloides poisoning. Clin Ter 1997;148:277–280. In Italian.

8. Mikos B, Biro E. Amanita phalloides poisoning in a 15-year case load of a pediatric intensive care unit. Orv Hetil 1993;134:907–910. In Hungarian.

9. Kacic M, Dujsin M, Puretic Z, Slavicek J. Mycetismus in children—report of an epidemic of poisoning. Lijec Vjesn 1990;112:369–373. In Serbo-Croatian (Roman).

10. Ghiringhelli L, Ceriani A, Lepore G, Moda S. Phallin syndrome. Reports on 28 cases. Minerva Med 1981;72:2499–2508. In Italian.

11. Langer M, Vesconi S, Iapichino G, Costantino D, Radrizzani D. The early removal of amatoxins in the treatment of amanita phalloides poisoning. Klin Wochenschr 1980;58:117–123. In German.

12. Costantino D, Damia G. Phalloidine intoxication. Results of various forms of treatment in 47 patients. Nouv Presse Med 1977;6:2315–2317. In French.

MUSHROOMS: CORTINARIUS

Cortinarius poisoning is caused by the bipyridyl toxins orellanine and orelline. Gastritis, chills, headaches, and myalgias may occur 1 day after ingestion. A small number of patients will develop acute renal failure in the form of tubulointerstitial nephritis (1). Delpech et al (2,3) reported the case of a deliberate ingestion of two raw carpophores of the mushroom *Cortinarius orellanus*. The patient was hospitalized 10 days later with acute renal failure (creatinine 1100 μmol/L). On admission, the plasma still contained orellanine. Management included six hemodialysis treatments, one TPE, and the administration of diltiazem and amino acids. Plasma and tissue assays of orellanine were performed by two-dimensional thin-layer chromatography. Eighteen months after the attempted suicide, the plasma creatinine level was 181 μmol/L. Although plasmapheresis was part of the successful management of this patient, the pharmacodynamic necessity for TPE is not clear.

REFERENCES

1. Brent J, Kulig K, Rumack BH. Mushrooms. In: Haddad LM, Winchester JF, eds. Clinical management of poisoning and drug overdose. 2nd ed. Philadelphia: WB Saunders, 1990:581–590.

2. Delpech N, Rapior S, Donnadieu P, Cozette AP, Ortiz JP, Huchard G. Voluntary poisoning by *Cortinarius orellanus*: useful-

ness of an original early treatment after determination of orellanine in the biological fluids and tissues. Nephrologie 1991;12:63–66. In French.
3. Delpech N, Rapior S, Cozette AP, Ortiz JP, Donnadieu P, Andary C, Huchard G. Outcome of acute renal failure caused by voluntary ingestion of *Cortinarius orellanus*. Presse Med 1990; 19:122–124. In French.

MUSHROOMS: *PAXILLUS INVOLUTUS*

Brown roll-rim (*Paxillus involutus*) is a dangerous poisonous mushroom with symptoms occurring a few hours after consumption. Repeated consumption may cause sensitization to a heat-stable toxin, resulting in hemolysis, whereas severe gastrointestinal symptoms may be due to a heat-instable toxin. Treatment for immune-mediated hemolysis consists of symptomatic therapy, corticosteroids, and possibly plasmapheresis (1).

REFERENCE

1. Olesen LL. Poisoning with the brown roll-rim mushroom, *Paxillus involutus*. Ugeskr Laeger 1991;153:445. In Danish.

PARAQUAT POISONING

Paraquat is a toxic herbicide that can cause renal failure, thus slowing its elimination. Tsatsakis et al (1) recently reported on 10 cases of acute paraquat poisoning in whom ultimate mortality was 50%. On admission (from 2 to 41 hours after ingestion), paraquat plasma levels varied from 0.4 to 6.0 µg/mL, whereas urine levels varied from 0.5 to 12.8 µg/mL. Besides standard supportive treatment, hemoperfusion hemodialysis and/or plasmapheresis were performed. The pharmacokinetic data confirmed considerable paraquat rebound from tissues to blood. Postmortem analysis showed substantial accumulation in kidney, lung, and liver (200 to 800 µg/g). Paraquat crossed the placenta and concentrated there to higher levels than in the mother's blood.

In an earlier report, a sublethal dose of paraquat poisoning was successfully managed with two TPE treatments approximating 2 liters per exchange (2). Although pre- and postpheresis levels suggested a substantial lowering of blood paraquat levels, the concomitant initiation of other therapies, including ingestion of activated charcoal and the ongoing excretion by normal renal function, made this report difficult to assess. In a critique of the authors' conclusions, Miller et al (3) pointed to the successful ability of hemodialysis to remove paraquat and that the relation between ongoing gastrointestinal absorption and renal excretion is the major factor dictating a need for extracorporeal therapy. Although worthy of further investigation, current recommendations suggest the use of hemoperfusion as a better documented removal technique (4).

REFERENCES

1. Tsatsakis AM, Perakis K, Koumantakis E. Experience with acute paraquat poisoning in Crete. Vet Hum Toxicol 1996;38:113–117.
2. Dearnaley DR, Martin MFR. Plasmapheresis for paraquat poisoning. Lancet 1978;1:162.
3. Miller J, Sanders E, Webb D. Plasmapheresis for paraquat poisoning. Lancet 1978;1:875–876. Letter.
4. Winchester JF. Paraquat and the bipyridyl herbicides. In: Haddad LM, Winchester JF, eds. Clinical management of poisoning and drug overdose. 2nd ed. Philadelphia: WB Saunders, 1990:1088–1103.

PARATHION POISONING

Methylparathion is an organophosphate pesticide that can block cholinesterase activity. The poison is lipid soluble and has a high affinity for serum proteins and is therefore not removed by dialysis or forced diuresis (1). A report involving three separate intoxications described the successful use of a plasmaperfusion technique for the removal of toxic levels (2). Removed plasma was perfused over activated charcoal and then returned to the patient. A 3.6-liter perfusion reduced methaphos levels from 33 to 8.8 μg/dL, a 3.2-liter perfusion lowered levels from 300 to 5.3 μg/dL, and a 7-liter perfusion reduced levels from 250 to 80 μg/dL. A reasonable assessment of this report would conclude that standard TPE with 3 to 7 liters of exchanged plasma, replaced with albumin, would likely produce the same degree of toxin removal.

REFERENCES

1. Wenz B, Barland P. Therapeutic intensive plasmapheresis. Semin Hematol 1981;18;147–162.

2. Luzhnikov EA, Yaroslavsky AA, Molodenkov MN, Surkalin BK, Evseev NG, Barsukov UF. Plasma perfusion through charcoal in methylparathion poisoning. Lancet 1977;1:38–39.

PHENYLBUTAZONE

TPE has been studied in animals as a means of removing the highly protein-bound phenylbutazone (98% protein bound). A single TPE equaling one blood volume or three TPE treatments equaling half of the blood volume each, performed at 20-minute intervals, significantly accelerated the elimination of phenylbutazone and resulted in 100% survival (1). A single plasmapheresis equaling three times the blood volume had the greatest effect in lowering the concentration of phenylbutazone in the blood, but only one of three animals survived (1).

REFERENCE

1. Lembeck F, Beubler E, Lepuschutz HF, Stolze A. Plasmapheresis in the elimination of toxic substances with marked plasma protein-binding properties. Wien Klin Wochenschr 1977;89: 257–260. In German.

PHENYTOIN

Phenytoin is widely used as an anticonvulsant. Intoxication results in ataxia, nystagmus, drowsiness, and behavioral abnormalities. Coma and respiratory depression are uncommon, and intoxication is rarely fatal despite substantial ingestion (100 to 160 mg/kg). Phenytoin's high protein binding makes it a poor candidate for hemodialysis, peritoneal dialysis, or hemoperfusion (1). Larsen et al. (2) reported a case of phenytoin intoxication in which a single 3-liter plasma exchange removed 107 mg of phenytoin. Although the treatment had minimal effect on serum levels, there appeared to be clinical improvement of mental status. In a previous attempt, three filter-based treatments involving from 2.5 to 3 liters each was capable of decreasing serum levels from 98 to 38 μg/mL (2). A report from Germany described the use of TPE in a 2-year-old boy experiencing coma after acute intoxication (3).

REFERENCES

1. Seger D. Phenytoin and other anticonvulsants. In: Haddad LM, Winchester JF, eds. Clinical management of poisoning and drug overdose. 2nd ed. Philadelphia: WB Saunders, 1990:877–893.
2. Larsen LS, Sterrett JR, Whitehead B, Marcus SM. Adjunctive therapy of phenytoin overdose—a case report using plasmaphoresis. J Toxicol Clin Toxicol 1986;24:37–49.
3. Scharf J, Ruder H, Harms D. Plasma separation in acute, intravenous phenytoin poisoning. Monatsschr Kinderheilkd 1990; 138:227–230. In German.

QUININE

Acute quinine toxicity can result in retinal damage and blindness. Previous reports suggested that plasma exchange may be a useful adjunct to enhancing drug removal (1,2). A comparison of net drug removal has been reported by Sabto et al (3) during an attempt to treat a 19-year-old man who had become blind from a quinine overdose. Serum level was 10.5 μg/mL 13 hours after ingestion. Forced diuresis was by far the most efficient method, removing 557 mg of quinine in 5 hours and a total of 1625 mg over 75 hours. A 6-hour hemodialysis removed 30 mg, 48 hours of peritoneal dialysis removed 1.6 mg/hr, and a 2-liter plasma exchange removed only 8.5 mg. The authors concluded that hemodialysis, peritoneal dialysis, and plasma exchange made only a minor contribution to quinine elimination by comparison with renal excretion. Current recommendations suggest that elimination by forced diuresis may be enhanced by urinary acidification with ammonium chloride or ascorbic acid (4).

REFERENCES

1. Dickinson P, Sabto J, West RH. Management of quinine toxicity. Trans Ophthalmol Soc N Z 1981;33:56–58.
2. Lockie P. Ocular toxicity of quinine. Med J Aust 1984;141:902.
3. Sabto JK, Pierce RM, West RH, Gurr FW. Hemodialysis, peritoneal dialysis, plasmapheresis and forced diuresis for the treatment of quinine overdose. Clin Nephrol 1981;16:264–268.
4. Compochiaro PA, Fogle JA, Spyker DA. Chemical and drug injury to the eye. In: Haddad LM, Winchester JF, eds. Clinical management of poisoning and drug overdose. 2nd ed. Philadelphia: WB Saunders, 1990:369–388.

SODIUM CHLORATE INTOXICATION

Sodium chlorate is a toxic constituent of certain herbicides. It is highly tissue bound and causes toxicity because of methemoglobin formation and renal failure partly resulting from hemolysis. TPE may be most useful as a means of removing free hemoglobin and red cell stroma (1,2). In one report, two successive daily TPE treatments exchanged a total of 7 liters of plasma with a resulting decline in free hemoglobin levels from 2.8 to 0.8 g/dL (3).

REFERENCES

1. Seyffart G. Plasmapheresis in treatment of acute intoxications. Trans Am Soc Artif Intern Organs 1982;28:673–676.
2. Jones JS, Dougherty J. Current status of plasmapheresis in toxicology. Ann Emerg Med 1986;15:474–482.
3. Davison AM, Mascie-Taylor BH, Robinson A, Barnard DL. The use of plasma exchange, transfusion and haemodialysis in the management of sodium chlorate intoxication. In: Sieberth HG, ed. Plasma exchange: plasmapheresis-plasmaseparation. Stuttgart: FK Schattauer Verlag, 1980:373–374.

THEOPHYLLINE

Theophylline toxicity manifests with cardiovascular and central nervous system toxicity. Because it is 55% protein bound and has a modest volume of distribution (0.4 to 0.7 L/kg), hemoperfusion has been considered a useful means of enhancing its removal (1). Multidose oral-activated charcoal is safe and effective but may be poorly tolerated in those with severe poisoning. Theophylline is also dialyzable and may be efficiently removed with a high-flux dialyzer and rapid blood flows, a technique that will also correct any eventual metabolic abnormalities. Laussen et al (2) reported on the use of arteriovenous and venovenous (pumped) plasma exchange in three children with theophylline toxicity, suggesting that plasmapheresis may be useful in increasing drug clearance and decreasing its half-life. Commentary on this report, however, pointed to several errors in the presentation of the data and suggested that proper evaluation of the efficacy of plasma exchange could not be made because endogenous clearance was not accounted for (3).

REFERENCES

1. Ehlers SM. Theophylline. In: Haddad LM, Winchester JF, eds. Clinical management of poisoning and drug overdose. 2nd ed. Philadelphia: WB Saunders, 1990:1407–1418.
2. Laussen P, Shann F, Butt W, Tibballs J. Use of plasmapheresis in acute theophylline toxicity. Crit Care Med 1991;19:288–290.
3. Jacobi J, Mowry JB. Use of plasmapheresis in acute theophylline toxicity. Crit Care Med 1992;20:151. Letter.

THYROXINE

Because thyroxine is highly protein bound, TPE has been used as a means of enhancing its removal after massive overdose. Despite rapid lowering of the serum levels immediately after each treatment, with an apparent shortening of half-lives (1), a pharmacokinetic analysis of the presented data suggests a rapid return to endogenous clearance rates after the procedure. A recent report provided serum and plasma extraction data in the immediate pre- and postpheresis period, demonstrating a rapid lowering of serum levels but an equally rapid rebound to pretreatment levels, suggesting that despite a reasonable removal of protein-bound drug, net removal of ingested drug by TPE is minimal (2). Thus, despite apparent success in the use of TPE for the treatment of endogenous thyrotoxicosis ("thyroid storm," see Graves' Disease and Thyroid Storm, Chap. 9), the usefulness of TPE treatment for exogenous thyrotoxicosis is not clear.

REFERENCES

1. Binimelis J, Bassas L, Marruecos L, Rodriguez J, Domingo ML, Madoz P, Armengol S, Mangues MA, de Leiva A. Massive thyroxine intoxication: evaluation of plasma extraction. Intensive Care Med 1987;13:33–38.
2. Henderson A, Hickman P, Ward G, Pond SM. Lack of efficacy of plasmapheresis in a patient overdosed with thyroxine. Anaesth Intensive Care 1994;22:463–464.

TRICYCLIC ANTIDEPRESSANTS

Intoxication with tricyclic antidepressants manifests with electrocardiographic abnormalities including T wave modifications, prolongation of QT interval, and bundle branch block (1). Ventricular dysrhythmia or myocardial failure suggests the most severe intoxications. Tricyclic antidepressants have an enormous volume of distribution, ranging from 6 to 50 L/g, or 420 to 3500 liters in a 70-kg patient. It is therefore not surprising that despite a high percentage of protein binding (92 to 97%), **neither hemoperfusion, TPE, nor hemodialysis has been found to be a useful means for net removal of drug (1)**. Despite one study that demonstrated a meager 2% elimination of ingested drug after 6 hours of hemoperfusion (2), there are anecdotal reports that suggest a rapid improvement in cardiotoxicity after hemoperfusion (3–5). Expert opinion is skeptical, however, because tricyclic antidepressant drug levels may spontaneously decrease rapidly after admission, presumably because of drug redistribution (6,7).

REFERENCES

1. Bouffard Y, Palmier B, Bouletreau P, Motin J. Acute tricyclic antidepressant intoxication. Evaluation of severity and treatment. A study of 16 patients with cardiovascular manifestations. Ann Med Interne (Paris) 1982;133:256–260. In French.
2. Pentel PR, Bullock ML, DeVane CL. Hemoperfusion for imipramine overdose: elimination of active metabolites. J Toxicol Clin Toxicol 1982;19:239–248.
3. Diaz-Buxo JA, Farmer CD, Chandler JT. Hemoperfusion in the treatment of amitriptyline intoxication. Trans Am Soc Artif Intern Organs 1978;24:699–703.
4. Marbury T, Mahoney J, Foller T, Juncos L, Cade R. Treatment of amitriptyline overdosage with charcoal hemoperfusion. Kidney Int 1978;12:485. Abstract.
5. Pedersen RS, Jorgensen KA, Olesen AS, Christensen KN. Charcoal haemoperfusion and antidepressant overdose. Lancet 1978;1:719–720. Letter.
6. Pentel PR, Keyler DE, Haddad LM. Tricyclic and newer antidepressants. In: Haddad LM, Winchester JF, eds. Clinical management of poisoning and drug overdose. 2nd ed. Philadelphia: WB Saunders, 1990:636–651.
7. Winchester JF. Poisoning: is the role of the nephrologist diminishing? Am J Kidney Dis 1989;13:171–183.

VINCRISTINE

Vincristine kinetics have a three-phase distribution, with an exponential phase lasting the first 5 minutes, a second phase lasting 1 to 2 hours, and a third phase lasting 85 hours. By the third phase, the volume of distribution is very large, estimated at 5 to 11 L/kg. Protein binding is about 75%. After an accidental overdose involving two 8-mg injections 12 hours apart, TPE exchanging 1.5 plasma volumes was performed 6 hours after the second dose and lowered concentrations from 7.1 to 5.5 ng/mL. Removed plasma contained 11.6 ng/mL. Twenty-four and 48 hours later, plasma concentrations were 2.3 and 2.1 ng/mL, respectively (1). Grade IV neutropenia lasted for only 4 days and neurologic toxicity was modest. A previous report of vincristine overdose in three children described successful treatment in two patients with double-volume exchange transfusion, prophylactic phenobarbital, and repetitive doses of folinic acid rescue (2).

REFERENCES

1. Pierga JY, Beuzeboc P, Dorval T, Palangie T, Pouillart P. Favourable outcome after plasmapheresis for vincristine overdose. Lancet 1992;340:185.
2. Kosmidis HV, Bouhoutsou DO, Varoutsi MC, Papadatos J, Stefanidis CG, Vlachos P, Scardoutsou A, Kostakis A. Vincristine overdose: experience with 3 patients. Pediatr Hematol Oncol 1991;8:171–178.

MISCELLANEOUS INTOXICATIONS

Single case reports described the use of TPE in several rare intoxications, including trichloroethylene (1), vanadate (2), and verapamil (3).

REFERENCES

1. Pelaia P, Volturo P, Sposato M, Conti G. A new therapeutic approach in the treatment of acute trichloroethylene poisoning. First clinical results. Minerva Anestesiol 1988;54:291–295. In Italian.

2. Schlake HP, Bertram HP, Husstedt IW, Schuierer G. Acute systemic vanadate poisoning presenting as cerebrovascular ischemia with prolonged reversible neurological deficits (PRIND). Clin Neurol Neurosurg 1994;96:92–95.
3. Siebenlist D. Plasma separation in verapamil poisoning. Dtsch Med Wochenschr 1990;115:797. Letter.

Therapeutic Cytapheresis

16

Leukapheresis   234
   Leukapheresis for Hyperleukocytosis   235
   Lymphocytapheresis for Rheumatoid Arthritis   236
Thrombopheresis   237
Erythrocytapheresis   238
   Erythrocytapheresis for Sickle Cell Disease   238
   Erythrocytapheresis for Babesiosis   239
   Erythrocytapheresis for Falciparum Malaria   239

A detailed review of cytapheresis is outside the scope of this book. Nonetheless, physicians who provide TPE may be called on to offer therapeutic options in certain conditions that have been found to be successfully treated with cytapheresis (1,2) (Table 16-1). This chapter provides a concise review of the current indications for therapeutic cytapheresis.

REFERENCES

1. Isbister JP. Cytapheresis: the first 25 years. Ther Apheresis 1997;1:17–21.
2. McLeod BC, Strauss RG, Ciavarella D, Gilcher RO, Kasprisin DO, Kiprov DD, Klein HG. Management of hematologic disorders and cancer. J Clin Apheresis 1993;8:211–230.

LEUKAPHERESIS

Leukapheresis may be useful for the treatment of the hyperviscosity syndrome associated with leukostasis, for the management of

Table 16-1.   Therapeutic Cytapheresis

	Reference and Year		
	1 **1986**	**2** **1993**	**3** **1994**
		Rating	
Therapeutic cytapheresis			
Leukapheresis			
Hyperleukocytosis syndrome	I	I	I
Leukemia without hyperleukocytosis syndrome	nl	nl	IV
Lymphocytopheresis for rheumatoid arthritis	II	III	III
Thrombopheresis			
Hyperviscosity/thrombotic crises	I	I	I
Erythrocytapheresis			
Sickle cell crises	I	I	I
Babesiosis	nl	nl	nl
Falciparum malaria	nl	nl	nl

Rating: I, standard therapy, acceptable but not mandatory; II, available evidence tends to favor efficacy: conventional therapy usually tried first; III, inadequately tested at this time; IV, no demonstrated value in controlled trials. nl, not listed.

REFERENCES: 1. American Medical Association Council on Scientific Affairs. Current status of therapeutic plasmapheresis. JAMA 1985;253:819–825.
2. Strauss RG, Ciavarella D, Gilcher RO, Kasprisin DO, Kiprov DD, Klein HG, McLeod BC. An overview of current management. J Clin Apheresis 1993;8:189–194.
3. Leitman SF, Ciavarella D, McLeod B, Owen H, Price T, Sniecinski I. Guidelines for therapeutic hemapheresis. Bethesda, MD: American Association of Blood Banks, revised 1994.

chronic myeloid leukemia during pregnancy, and for chronic lymphoid leukemia if conventional therapy has failed or is contraindicated (1). Lymphocytapheresis has been found to be useful in the management of rheumatoid arthritis.

Leukapheresis for Hyperleukocytosis

A hyperviscosity syndrome associated with large numbers of circulating blasts is manifested by headache, dizziness, altered mental status, and pulmonary insufficiency. Blasts of the monocytic, myelocytic, or myelomonocytic cell lines are considered the "stickiest," resulting in leukostasis, vascular occlusion, and perivascular leukemic infiltration. Release of lysosomal contents can initiate the coagulation cascade, causing catastrophic microvascular coagulation.

Involvement of the pulmonary circulation, resulting in acute respiratory distress syndrome, is a major complication. Given that chemotherapy may require a prolonged period before becoming effective, peripheral leukocytosis of 100×10^9/L may be temporarily managed with high-volume (>10 liters) leukapheresis. Daily treatments may be necessary until production of blasts can be controlled. An erythrocyte sedimentation agent such as hydroxyethyl starch is recommended to improve white blood cell (WBC) harvest and return of red cells (2).

In the pediatric population, leukapheresis has been shown to be effective as a cytoreductive procedure before the initiation of chemotherapy and as a treatment for pulmonary symptoms believed to be secondary to leukostasis (3). Nonetheless, childhood hyperleukocytosis has been successfully managed with intravenous hydration, urinary alkalinization, and allopurinol, providing a median reduction in WBC count of 81% (range, 66 to 98.8%) within a median period of 36 hours (range, 12 to 60 hours) (4).

A recent retrospective review demonstrated a lack of correlation between the degree of leucoreduction and early mortality (5). In 48 procedures, leukapheresis reduced pretreatment leukocyte counts by more than 50% and resulted in postapheresis WBC counts of less than 100×10^9/L in 65% of patients treated. Unfortunately, those patients presenting with neurologic, respiratory, or renal complications had higher early mortality rates than those without such complications, despite similar initial leukocyte counts and comparable leucoreductions.

Lymphocytapheresis for Rheumatoid Arthritis

In 1977, Paulus et al (6) demonstrated that lymphocyte depletion via a surgically created fistula in the thoracic duct was capable of decreasing the number of tender joints and decreasing the duration of morning stiffness in patients with rheumatoid arthritis. Subsequently, two randomized controlled studies using lymphapheresis as a means of lymphocyte depletion demonstrated similar benefit in reducing articular involvement (7,8) (Table 11-2). Despite this medical success, the use of lymphocytapheresis for rheumatoid arthritis has been limited by its costs and the limited duration of its effectiveness (see Chap. 11).

REFERENCES

1. Isbister JP. Cytapheresis: the first 25 years. Ther Apheresis 1997;1:17–21.

2. McLeod BC, Strauss RG, Ciavarella D, Gilcher RO, Kasprisin DO, Kiprov DD, Klein HG. Management of hematologic disorders and cancer. J Clin Apheresis 1993;8:211–230.
3. Bunin NJ, Kunkel K, Callihan TR. Cytoreductive procedures in the early management in cases of leukemia and hyperleukocytosis in children. Med Pediatr Oncol 1987;15:232–235.
4. Basade M, Dhar AK, Kulkarni SS, Sastry PS, Yadav RP, Parikh BS, Pai SK, Nair CN, Kurkure PA, Advani SH. Rapid cytoreduction in childhood leukemic hyperleukocytosis by conservative therapy. Med Pediatr Oncol 1995;25:204–207.
5. Porcu P, Danielson CF, Orazi A, Heerema NA, Gabig TG, McCarthy LJ. Therapeutic leukapheresis in hyperleucocytic leukaemias: lack of correlation between degree of cytoreduction and early mortality rate. Br J Haematol 1997;98:433–436.
6. Paulus HE, Machleder HI, Levine S, Yu DT, MacDonald NS. Lymphocyte involvement in rheumatoid arthritis. Arthritis Rheum 1977;20:1249–1262.
7. Karsh J, Klippel JH, Plotz PH, Decker JL, Wright DG, Flye MW. Lymphapheresis in rheumatoid arthritis: a randomized trial. Arthritis Rheum 1981;24:867–873.
8. Wallace DJ, Goldfinger D, Lowe C, Nichols S, Weiner J, Brachman M, Klinenberg JR. Double blind sham controlled trial of lymphoplasmapheresis versus sham pheresis in rheumatoid arthritis. N Engl J Med 1982;306:1406–1410.

THROMBOPHERESIS

Although previously reported to be occasionally effective for chronic management (1), thrombopheresis is most often a temporizing procedure that may be indicated in those patients with extreme elevations of thrombocytes ($>1000 \times 10^9$/L) who are manifesting signs of microvascular thrombosis or excessive bleeding (2–5). For those with signs of microvascular occlusion (hyperviscosity syndrome), the risk of platelet activation in the extracorporeal circuit should be considered and antiplatelet agents should be given. Dextran 70 or 40 as replacement fluid and low-molecular-weight heparin (less platelet activation than standard heparin) are recommended (3). Daily treatments may be required until peripheral counts are reduced or there is a substantial improvement in hyperviscosity-associated symptoms.

There may also be a role for thrombopheresis in pregnant women who are at risk of first-trimester abortions, intrauterine growth retardation, abruptio placentae, and premature delivery (3,6).

It should be noted that conventional therapy has been found to be very useful and that hydroxyurea has been effective in reducing thrombotic complications. Other effective treatments include alkylating agents, recombinant interferon alfa, and anagrelide (7). Antiplatelet therapy is most effective in patients with digital or cerebrovascular ischemic problems.

REFERENCES

1. Panlilio AL, Reiss RF. Therapeutic plateletpheresis in thrombocythemia. Transfusion 1979;19:147–152.
2. Taft EG, Babcock RB, Scharfman WB, Tartaglia AP. Plateletpheresis in the management of thrombocytosis. Blood 1977;50:927–933.
3. Isbister JP. Cytapheresis: the first 25 years. Ther Apheresis 1997; 1:17–21.
4. McLeod BC, Strauss RG, Ciavarella D, Gilcher RO, Kasprisin DO, Kiprov DD, Klein HG. Management of hematologic disorders and cancer. J Clin Apheresis 1993;8:211–230.
5. Adami R. Therapeutic thrombocytapheresis: a review of 132 patients. Int J Artif Organs Suppl 1993;5:183–184.
6. Eliyahu S, Shalev E. Essential thrombocythemia during pregnancy. Obstet Gynecol Surv 1997;52:243–247.
7. Schafer AI. Management of thrombocythemia. Curr Opin Hematol 1996;3:341–346.

ERYTHROCYTAPHERESIS

Erythrocyte removal with a blood separator offers the possibility of normovolemic reduction in hematocrit for patients with polycythemia vera, but most of these patients can be successfully treated with venesection alone (1). At present, the benefit of erythrocytapheresis is best appreciated for those conditions in which the entire red cell mass is either diseased or infested. Such is the case during episodes of severe microvascular occlusion associated with sickle cell disease (2), plasmodium falciparum, and babesiosis.

Erythrocytapheresis for Sickle Cell Disease

Erythrocytapheresis has been used to control sickle cell crises (3) and can be performed in an extremely efficient manner, allowing a 50% exchange in an adult within 2 hours (4). Kleinman et al (5) reviewed their experience with erythrocytapheresis in nine patients. Those patients with dangerous complications of sickle cell disease such as acute respiratory distress and priapism responded to erythrocytapheresis with marked improvement within 24 to 48 hours. Those with prolonged painful vaso-occlusive crises showed only variable improvement, whereas those treated to decrease the frequency of painful crises experienced no prolongation in symptom-free intervals. These authors concluded that erythrocytapheresis had its main value in the management of acute dangerous complications of sickle cell disease.

Erythrocytapheresis for Babesiosis

Babesiosis is a malaria-like parasitic disease that is most often associated with mild illness. Machtinger et al (6) reported a case of severe babesiosis in a human immunodeficiency virus–positive splenectomized man in whom red blood cell exchange transfusion resulted in prompt and sustained (26 months) clinical improvement. Red blood cell exchange transfusion, combined with antibiotic therapy, appears to be a rapidly effective therapeutic modality that can induce rapid and sustained remissions.

Erythrocytapheresis for Falciparum Malaria

Despite the lack of well-designed clinical trials, exchange transfusion has been recommended as an adjunct to the treatment of severe falciparum malaria. Aquinas et al (7) reported that a 4-unit exchange transfusion resulted in prompt clinical improvement and a reduction in parasitemia. These results suggest that erythrocytapheresis may offer a therapeutically efficient means for providing clinical improvement in the management of drug-resistant malaria.

REFERENCES

1. Isbister JP. Cytapheresis: the first 25 years. Ther Apheresis 1997;1:17–21.
2. McLeod BC, Strauss RG, Ciavarella D, Gilcher RO, Kasprisin DO, Kiprov DD, Klein HG. Management of hematologic disorders and cancer. J Clin Apheresis 1993;8:211–230.
3. Green M, Hall RJ, Huntsman RG, Lawson A, Pearson TC, Wheeler PC. Sickle cell crisis treated by exchange transfusion. Treatment of two patients with heterozygous sickle cell syndrome. JAMA 1975;231:948–950.

4. Klein HG, Garner RJ, Miller DM, Rosen SL, Statham NJ, Winslow RM. Automated partial exchange transfusion in sickle cell anemia. Transfusion 1980;20:578–584.
5. Kleinman SH, Hurvitz CG, Goldfinger D. Use of erythrocyta-pheresis in the treatment of patients with sickle cell anemia. J Clin Apheresis 1984;2:170–176.
6. Machtinger L, Telford SR III, Inducil C, Klapper E, Pepkowitz SH, Goldfinger D. Treatment of babesiosis by red blood cell exchange in an HIV-positive, splenectomized patient. J Clin Apheresis 1993;8:78–81.
7. Aquinas S, Ross C, Vincent J, Sridhar CB. Partial exchange trans-fusion in the treatment of severe falciparum malaria. Natl Med J India 1996;9:163–165.

Index

Acetylcholine blockage, 102–103
Acetylsalicylic acid removal, 81
Agglutinins, 134
Albumin
  advantage and disadvantages of, 29
  anaphylactic reactions to, 30
  colloid oncotic pressure of, 29
  depletion coagulopathy with, 30
  distribution and metabolism of, 9t
  electrolyte composition of, 29
  immunoglobulin depletion with,
    30
  as replacement fluid, 28–31
    for anti-GBM antibody-mediated
      disease, 181
    coagulation factor depletion with,
      62
    in hyperviscosity syndrome, 112
    for peripheral neuropathy in HIV
      patients, 211
    postpheresis infection and, 64–65
    reactions to, 69–70
  serum, 69
  viral transmission via, 31
Alkalosis, 33, 72
Alkylating agents, 238
Aluminum, accumulation of, 72–73
Amanita phalloides poisoning, 222–223
Amanita verna poisoning, 222–223
Aminoglycoside removal, 80
Amniocentesis, for maternal-fetal

incompatibility, 136
Amyotrophic lateral sclerosis
  indication for TPE, 89–90
  treatment of, 104
Anagrelide, 238
Anaphylactic/anaphylactoid reactions
  to ACE inhibitors, 71
  to albumin solution, 30
  to fresh frozen plasma, 33
  incidence of, 53
  to protein-containing replacement
    fluids, 69–70
  treatment of, 33, 69–70
Anemia
  autoimmune hemolytic
    cold agglutinin-mediated, 134
    warm agglutinin-mediated,
      134–135
  management of, 62
  with plasma exchange, 60–62
Angiotensin-converting enzyme (ACE)
    inhibitors
  anaphylactoid reactions to, 49–50
  atypical reactions to, 71
  with fresh frozen plasma, 34
  with Prosorba column
    immunoadsorption, 47–48
Antecubital veins, for hemoaccess,
    36–37
Anti-acetylcholine receptor (AChR)
    antibodies, 94–95

241

Antibodies, stimulating pathogenic
    production of, 15–16
Anticardiolipin antibodies, 163
Anticoagulants, 165
Anticoagulation
  with dialysis equipment, 25
  in TPE, 26–28
Anti-GBM antibody-mediated disease,
    180–181
Anti-GBM-associated disease, 182–183
    treatment of, 185
Anti-glomerular basement membrane
    antibody, 15
Antihistamines, 145
Anti-HLA antibodies, 195–196
Antimyeloperoxidase antibodies,
    167–168
Antineutrophil cytoplasmic
    autoantibodies (ANCA)
  positivity for, 180
  in scleroderma, 167–168
Antineutrophil cytoplasmic
    autoantibody (ANCA)-
    associated disease, 183
  vasculitis and, 172–173
Antiphospholipid antibody syndrome,
    163–164, 178–179
Antiplatelet therapy
  of digital or cerebrovascular
      ischemia, 238
  for thrombotic thrombocytopenic
      purpura, 118
Antithrombin III
  distribution and metabolism of, 9t
  post-treatment depletion of, 62
  serum levels after plasma exchange,
      59
Apheresis Instrumentation, 20–21
Apneic events, 74
Apoprotein B lipoprotein removal,
    selective, 49–50
Arrhythmia, hypokalemic, 72
Arsine poisoning, 217
Arteriovenous access, permanent, 37, 41
Arteriovenous fistula
  primary, 41

surgical replacement of, 37
Arteriovenous graft, permanent
    vascular fistula in, 41
ASA, volume of distribution of, 80t
Aspartate amino transferase, 124
Aspiration, for catheter clotting, 38
AT-III. *See* Antithrombin III
Autoantibodies
  to insulin receptor, 149
  pathogenic, removal of, 3–4
  prolonged suppression of, 16
Autoimmune neuropathy, 210–211
Azathioprine
  for bullous pemphigoid, 154
  for chronic inflammatory
      demyelinating polyneuropathy,
      96–97
  for Eaton-Lambert syndrome, 103
  for rapidly progressive
      glomerulonephritis, 183–184
  removal during TPE, 80

Babesiosis, 239
Beta-carotene, removal of, 73
Biocompatible membranes, reducing
    adverse reactions, 74
Blood flow rate, 24f
  for citrate solution-to-whole blood
      ratios, 27t
Blood purification techniques, 216
  conditions for, 3
Bradykinin metabolism disorder, 141
Bullous pemphigoid, 154
Burn shock, 205

C3, distribution and metabolism of,
    9t
C4, distribution and metabolism of,
    9t
Calcium
  for citrate-induced paresthesia, 56
  ionized, in centrifugal techniques,
      26–27
  kinetics of with and without
      supplemental infusion, 57t
Calcium channel antibodies, 102–103

Campylobacter jejuni, 91
Candida infection, 38
Cannulation, femoral vein, 39
Carbamazepine poisoning, 218
Cascade filtration, 43–44
Cast nephropathy
  controlled study of TPE for, 189t
  treatment of, 187–188
Catastrophic antiphospholipid
    syndrome, 163, 164
Catheters
  clotting of, 38
  large-bore double-lumen, 39
  percutaneous or implanted, 37
  radiologic evaluation of placement
    of, 40
  temporary vascular
    femoral vein cannulation, 39
    infection control in, 37–38
    internal jugular, 40
    maintaining patency of, 38–39
    subclavian, 40
    tunneled jugular, 40
Cefazolin, 80t
Cefotetan, 80t
Ceftriaxone, 80t
Cellular components, return to patient
    of, 19
Cellulose diacetate membrane, 24
Central nervous system lupus, 89
Centrifugation, 18
  citrate infusions in, 26–27
  systems for, 19–20
Cerebral ischemia, 62
Chemotherapy
  for hyperviscosity syndrome, 113
  for renal failure with multiple
    myeloma, 187–188
Chlorambucil, 113
Chlorhexidine, 38
2-Chlorodeoxyadenosine, 113
Chlorpropamide, 80t
Cholestasis, 144–145
Cholesterol
  distribution and metabolism of, 9t
  high-density-lipoprotein (HDL),

selective removal of, 49–50
low-density lipoprotein (LDL)
  lowering of, 49
  lowering serum levels of, 141–142
Cholesterol-containing lipoproteins,
    removal of, 3
Cholestyramine, 145
Cholinesterase, reduced levels of, 74
Churg-Strauss syndrome, 172
  treatment of, 173–174
Cirrhosis, primary biliary, 141–142
Cisplatin poisoning, 218–219
Citrate
  hypocalcemia with, 56–58
  toxicity of, 25, 56, 58
    with fresh frozen plasma, 33
Citrate anticoagulation, 19
  with centrifugal devices, 25
Citrate infusions
  in centrifugal techniques, 26–27
  dosage of, 27
Citrate solutions
  maximum blood flow rates and, 27t
  solute content of, 28t
Citrate-induced alkalemia, 33
Coagulation abnormalities, 59–62
Coagulation factors
  depletion of with albumin solution,
    30
  inability to produce, 145–146
  post-treatment depletion of, 62
  serum levels after plasma exchange,
    59t
Coagulopathy
  depletion, 43, 59–60
    with albumin solution, 30
    with hemophilia treatment,
      137–138
    with lupus-related renal disease,
      165
  post-treatment, 60–61f
Cold agglutinins, 134
Colestipol, 145
Colloid oncotic pressure, 29
Colloid solution, starch-based, 35–36
Coma, hepatic, 146

Complications
  incidence of, 53–54
  prevalence of, 53–54
  specific, 56–77
Continuous flow system, 19–20
Corticosteroids
  for chronic inflammatory
    demyelinating polyneuropathy,
    96–97
  for *Paxillus involutus* poisoning, 225
  for pemphigus vulgaris, 152
  for thrombotic thrombocytopenic
    purpura, 118
Cortinarius poisoning, 224
CREST syndrome, 166
Cryofiltration, 45
Cryoglobulinemia
  nephritis-associated, 178–179
  treatment of, 99, 114–116
  types of, 114
Cryoglobulinemic polyneuropathy, 89
Cryoglobulins, 114
  removal of, 3
Cryosupernatant, 121
Cyclophosphamide
  for chronic inflammatory
    demyelinating polyneuropathy,
    96–97
  for hemophilia, 138
  for hyperviscosity syndrome, 113
  for rapidly progressive
    glomerulonephritis, 183–184
  removal during TPE, 79–80
  for renal failure with multiple
    myeloma, 187
  for vasculitis, 173–174
Cyclosporin A, 96–97
Cytapheresis, 18
  indications for, 234–239
Cytokines
  circulating, 197
  endotoxin-initiated, 198–199
Cytotoxic antibodies, 195–196

Danazol, 129
Death, treatment-associated, 54

Depletion syndromes, with cascade
    filtration, 43–44
Dermatologic disorders
  indicating TPE, 86t
  treatment of, 151–158
Dermatomyositis, 175
Dextran sulfate
  anaphylactoid reactions to, 49–50
  for selective lipid removal, 49–50
Dialysis
  equipment for, 23–24
    anticoagulation and, 25
    operating parameters for, 24–25
    in plasma exchange, 18
    vascular access in, 25
  for renal failure with multiple
    myeloma, 189
Diclofenac, 80t
Dicloxacillin, 80t
Digitoxin
  overdose of, 220
  removal during TPE, 81
Digoxin, removal of, 81
Digoxin-specific antibody fragments,
    221
Diltiazem overdose, 221–222
Diphenhydramine
  with fresh frozen plasma, 33
  for reactions to protein-containing
    replacement fluids, 69–70
Diuresis, 228
Drugs
  kinetics of, 78
  removal during TPE, 78–81

Eaton-Lambert syndrome
  cause of, 102–103
  indication for TPE, 89
  treatment of, 103
ECV. *See* Extracorporeal volume
Eicosanoids, 197
Electrolytes
  abnormalities of, 72–73
  in albumin solutions, 29
Encephalomyelitis, acute disseminated
    (ADEM)

indicating TPE, 89
treatment of, 105
Endotoxemia, 201–203
Endotoxic shock, 201
Endotoxins
adsorption of, 52
in fulminant systemic
meningococcemia, 198–199
removal of, 3
selective removal of, 197
in septic syndromes, 201–203
End-stage renal disease, 180
Enzyme replacement therapy, 108
Ephedrine, 70
Epinephrine, 70
EPV. See Estimated plasma volume
(EPV)
Erythrocytapheresis
for babesiosis, 239
for falciparum malaria, 239
indications for, 238
for sickle cell disease, 238–239
Escherichia coli 0157-H7 verotoxin, 125
Estimated plasma volume (EPV), 5
calculation of, 6–7
by weight and hematocrit, 6t
Exchange transfusion
double-volume, 232
Exchange volume, calculation of, 6–7
Excorim protein A system, 46, 48–49
Extracorporeal blood purification
techniques
endotoxin adsorption by, 52
rationale for, 3–4
Extracorporeal circuit, 26–28
Extracorporeal volume, 19

Factor VIII
distribution and metabolism of, 9t
inhibitors of, removing, 137–138
Falciparum malaria, 239
Fat overload syndrome, 144
Femoral vein cannulation, 39
Fetal loss, recurrent with, 163–164
Fetal sampling, 136
FFP. See Fresh frozen plasma

Fibrinogen
distribution and metabolism of, 9t
serum levels after plasma exchange,
59
Filtration, 21–22
double, 43–44
double cascade, 50, 115
Folinic acid rescue, 232
Fresh frozen plasma
AIDS-related complex, 209–210
anaphylactoid reactions to, 33
incidence of, 53
for anti-GBM antibody-mediated
disease, 181
citrate toxicity and, 33
components of, 32
death associated with, 76–77
for fulminant systemic
meningococcemia, 199
for HELLP syndrome, 124
for hemophilia, 138
for hepatic failure, 146
infection with, 63–66
for myasthenia gravis, 94
versus plasma protein fraction, 34
for porphyria cutanea tarda, 156–157
for post-transfusion purpura, 133
potential problems of, 32–33
reactions to, 69–70
for thrombotic thrombocytopenic
purpura, 119–121
viral transmission with, 33–34
Fulminant systemic meningococcemia,
198
treatment of, 199–200

G forces, 19
Giant cell arteritis, 172
Glomerulonephritis
immunologically based, 178
indication for TPE, 178–196
infection postpheresis, 64
rapidly progressive, 172–173,
182–183
treatment of, 183–185
in scleroderma, 168

Glomerulosclerosis, focal segmental, 192–193
Glyburide, 80t
Goodpasture's syndrome, 15. See also Anti-GBM antibody-mediated disease
Granulocyte macrophage colony-stimulating factor, 219
Graves' disease
  ophthalmopathy in, 148–149
  treatment of, 147–148
Guillain-Barré syndrome
  indication for TPE, 89
  Study Group, 92t
  treatment of, 91–93

HELLP syndrome
  catastrophic antiphospholipid syndrome and, 164
  differential diagnosis of, 123–124
  in pregnancy, 122–123
  treatment of, 124
HELP system, 49
Hematologic disorders
  indication for TPE, 86t
  treatment of, 110–138
Hemodialysis
  drug kinetics during, 78
  porphyria cutanea tarda and, 156
  for tricyclic overdose, 231
Hemofiltration
  convection-based, 189
  for hepatic failure, 146, 189
Hemolytic-uremic syndrome, 179
  in adults, 125–126
  in children, 128
  fresh frozen plasma for, 32–33
  in HIV patients, 209–210
  mitomycin-induced cancer-associated, 125–126
  in pregnancy, 122–123
  recurrent in renal transplantation, 126
Hemoperfusion, 229
Hemophilia, 137–138
Hemorrhage, 33

Henoch-Schönlen purpura, 190–191
Heparin
  with membrane plasma separation, 25
  volume of distribution of, 80t
Hepatic failure, 145–146
Hepatitis A, 146
Hepatitis B
  with fresh frozen plasma, 33–34
  with plasma exchange, 65
Hepatitis C
  with fresh frozen plasma, 34
  with plasma exchange, 65
  transmitted by albumin preparation, 31
Hepatitis infection, 31–34, 65, 146
Hollow fiber, section of, 21f
Human immunodeficiency virus (HIV)
  accidental transmission to patients and staff of, 208–209
  with fresh frozen plasma, 34
  immunodepression in, 207–208
  indication for TPE, 87t
  with plasma exchange, 65
  syndromes of, 206
  therapeutic plasma exchange in patients with, 206–211
Human T-cell lymphotropic virus (HTLV)
  with fresh frozen plasma, 34
  with plasma exchange, 65
Hydroxyurea, 238
Hypercholesterolemia
  familial, 140–141
  in primary biliary cirrhosis, 141–142
  treatment of, 139–141
Hyperleukocytosis, 235–236
Hypertriglyceridemia, 144
Hyperviscosity syndrome
  characteristics of, 110–111
  leukapheresis for, 234–235
  with macroglobulinemia, 98
  in rheumatoid vasculitis, 171
  treatment of, 112–113
Hypocalcemia

with centrifugal techniques, 27
citrate-induced, 56–58
Hypocomplementemia, filter-related, 74
Hypokalemia, postpheresis, 72
Hypo-oncotic replacement solution, 75
Hypotension, 75–76
Hypothermia, 74
Hypovolemia, hypo-oncotic, 75–76

Ibuprofen, 80t
IgA nephropathy, 190–191
IgA synthesis, dysregulation of, 190–191
IgG
    half-life of, 3
    maternal-fetal transfer of, 136
    pathogenic antibodies and, 15
    progressive decline in pretreatment serum concentrations of, 10f
IgG antibodies, adsorption of, 46–47
IgG-containing immune complexes, 185
IgM
    in hyperviscosity syndrome, 110–111
    progressive decline in pretreatment serum concentrations of, 11f
Immune complexes, removal of, 3
Immune-based disorders, 207–208, 209
Immunoadsorbent system, 49–50
Immunoadsorbent techniques
    Excorim, 46, 48–49
    IMRE Prosorba column, 46–48
    protein A, 45–46, 137–138, 192–193
Immunoadsorption, 137–138
    indications for, 46t
Immunoglobulin. See also Cryoglobulins
    apheresis-induced deficiency of, 181
    decline in levels versus total body load of, 14–15
    depletion of with albumin solution, 30
    disordered production of, 186
    distribution and metabolism of, 9t

extravascular distribution of, 8–9
intravenous infusion of, 30
    viral transmission via, 31
intravenous (IVIG)
    for Guillain-Barré syndrome, 92–93
    for hemophilia, 138
    in HIV patients, 208
    for idiopathic thrombocytopenic purpura, 129
    for postpheresis infection, 65
    for post-transfusion purpura, 133
kinetics of removal of, 13–16
long half-lives of, 14
removal as result of plasma exchange, 8f
serum decline after TPE, 8–10
serum levels with plasma exchange, 64
Immunomodulation therapy, 130–131
Immunosuppression, postpheresis, 16
Immunosuppressive agents
    for chronic inflammatory demyelinating polyneuropathy, 96–97
    for idiopathic thrombocytopenic purpura, 129
    for lupus-related renal disease, 165
    for pemphigus vulgaris, 152–153
    for rapidly progressive glomerulonephritis, 183–184
    for sensorineural hearing loss, 106–107
    for vasculitis, 174
IMRE Prosorba column, 46–48
Indications, 86–88t. See also specific indications
Indomethacin, 80t
Infection
    control of in temporary vascular catheters, 37–38
    with plasma exchange, 63–66
    postpheresis, 64–65
Inflammatory mediators, endotoxin-initiated, 198–199
Inflammatory processes, 52

Inner ear disease, immune-mediated, 106–107
Insulin receptor autoantibodies, 149
Intensive care unit (ICU), TPE indications in, 197–205
Interferon alfa, 116
  recombinant, for thrombotic complications of thrombocytosis, 238
Intoxications
  guidelines for use of TPE for, 215–216
  indication for TPE, 87–88t, 214–232
Intravenous fat emulsion administration, 144
Iodine, 147
Isaacs' syndrome, 105
IVIG. See Immunoglobulin, intravenous (IVIG)

Jugular catheters, 40

Ketorolac, 80t
Kinin formation, 33

Large-molecular-weight substances
  absorption rate of, 5–6
  extravascular distribution of, 8–9
Leukapheresis
  for hyperleukocytosis, 235–236
  indications for, 234–235
  for polymyositis and dermatomyositis, 175
  for rheumatoid arthritis, 236
Leukemia
  chronic myeloid, 235
  lymphoid, 235
Leukocytopenia, filter-related, 74
Light chains
  limiting synthesis of, 188
  removal of, 189
  in renal failure, 186–188
  in serum and urine, 188f
Lipids. See also Cholesterol; Lipoproteins
Lipids, selective removal of, 49–50

Lipoproteins. See also Cholesterol
  distribution and metabolism of, 9t
  low-density (LDL)
    extracorporeal precipitation of, 49
    precipitation of, 141
Liposorba system, 50
Lupus anticoagulant, 163, 178–179
  renal disease and, 164–165
Lupus-related morbidities, 160–161, 163–165
Lyell's syndrome. See Toxic epidermal necrolysis
Lymphapheresis, 169–170
Lymphocytapheresis, 235
  for rheumatoid arthritis, 169–170
Lymphocyte clones, 3
Lymphocyte depletion, 169
Lymphoplasmapheresis
  for rheumatoid arthritis, 169–170
  for scleroderma, 166–167

Maternal-fetal incompatibility, 136
Melphalan, 187
Membrane
  cellulose diacetate, 24
  permeability of, 22f
  pore sizes of, 21
Membrane plasma separation, 18, 21–22. See also Filtration
  anticoagulation in, 25
  with dialysis equipment, 23–25
  operating parameters of, 24–25
  vascular access in, 25
Meningococcemia, 201–203
Metabolic alkalosis, 72
  with fresh frozen plasma, 33
Metabolic disorders
  indication for TPE, 86t
  treatment of, 139–149
Methimazole, 147
Methylparathion poisoning, 226
Methylprednisolone, 154
Minocycline, 38
Mitomycin-induced cancer-associated hemolytic-uremic syndrome, 125–126

Monoclonal antibodies, 98
Monoclonal gammopathy of
    undetermined significance,
    98
Multiple myeloma, 179
  renal failure in, 186–189
    treatment of, 187–189
Multiple sclerosis
  indication for TPE, 89
  pathogenesis of, 100
  treatment of, 100–101
Muscle cramps, 53
Mushroom poisoning, 222–223, 224,
    225
Myasthenia gravis
  IgG level and, 15
  indication for TPE, 89
  treatment of, 94–95
Myeloma cast nephropathy, 187–188
Myeloma light chains, removal of, 3
Myocardial infarction, 62

Naloxone, 145
Naproxen, 80t
Neurologic disorders, 86t, 89–90
Neuromyotonia
  indication for TPE, 89
  treatment of, 105
Neurotoxins, failure to detoxify,
    145–146
Niklasson prognostic scores, 198, 199
Nikolsky's sign, 151
Nitric oxide, 197
  endotoxin-initiated, 198–199

Ophthalmopathy, Graves', 148–149
Orellanine, 224
Orelline, 224
Organophosphate pesticide poisoning,
    226

Paraneoplastic syndromes, 89–90
Paraquat poisoning, 225–226
Parathion poisoning, 226
Paresthesia, citrate-induced, 53, 56
Partial thromboplastin time (PTT)

after plasma exchange, 59
  change in, 60–61f
Paxillus involutus poisoning, 225
Pemphigus vulgaris
  diagnosis of, 151–152
  features of, 151
  treatment of, 152–153
Peripheral neuropathy
  in cryoglobulinemia, 99
  in HIV patients, 210–211
  in hyperviscosity syndrome, 112–113
  in rheumatoid vasculitis, 171
Phenobarbital
  for cholestasis-induced pruritus, 145
  removal during TPE, 79t
  for vincristine overdose, 232
Phenylbutazone poisoning, 227
Phenytoin
  removal of, 79t, 80–81
  toxicity of, 227
Phlebotomy, 156
Photopheresis
  for renal allograft rejection, 194
  for scleroderma, 167
Phytanic acid, 107, 108
Plasma
  filtration rates of, 24f
  flow rate of versus blood flow, 24f
  infusion, for thrombotic
      thrombocytopenic purpura,
      119–121
  protein fraction of, 34
    reactions to, 69–70
  proteins, distribution and metabolism
      of, 9t
  separation of, 19. *See also* Membrane
      plasma separation
    by filtration, 21–22
Plasma exchange. *See* Therapeutic
    plasma exchange
Plasma reactive antibodies (PRA), 195–
    196
Plasmaflo filter
  operating parameters of, 24–25
  permeability of, 22f
  plasma filtration rates with, 24f

Plasmaperfusion, 226
Plasmapheresis. *See also* Therapeutic
    plasma exchange
  for anti-GBM antibody-mediated
    disease, 180–181
  for anti-GBM-associated disease, 185
  for cisplatin overdose, 219
  complications of, 53, 54t
  for cortinarius poisoning, 224
  for cryoglobulinemia, 114–116
  death associated with, 76–77
  for hemophilia, 137
  for hyperviscosity syndrome, 112–113
  indications for, 86–87t
  for *Paxillus involutus* poisoning, 225
  for phenylbutazone poisoning, 227
  for post-transplant focal segmental
    glomeruloscerlosis, 193
  for Raynaud's disease, 176
  for renal allograft rejection, 193–194
  for renal failure with multiple
    myeloma, 187
  for rheumatoid arthritis, 169–170
  for scleroderma, 168
  selective techniques, 42–43
Polyarteritis, microscopic, 172
Polyarteritis nodosa, 172
  hepatitis B-associated, 173–174
  treatment of, 173–174
Polymyositis, 175
Polymyxin B hemoperfusion, 203
Polyneuropathy
  associated with monoclonal
    gammopathies, 89
  chronic inflammatory demyelinating
    indication for TPE, 89
    treatment of, 96–97
  paraprotein-associated
    cryoglobulinemia, 99
    monoclonal gammopathy of
      undetermined significance, 98
    Waldenström's macroglobulinemia,
      98–99
Porphyria cutanea tarda, 156–157
Post-transfusion purpura, 133
Prednisolone

for rapidly progressive
    glomerulonephritis, 183–184
  removal during TPE, 79
Prednisone
  for Eaton-Lambert syndrome, 103
  removal during TPE, 79
Pregnancy
  thrombopheresis during, 237–238
  TTP in, 122–123
Probenecid, 80t
Propranolol, removal of, 81
Propylthiouracil, 147
Prostacyclin, 118–119
Protein A immunoadsorption column,
    45–46
  for hemophilia, 137–138
  for post-transplant focal segmental
    glomeruloscerlosis, 192–193
Protein-binding drugs, 80t
Prothrombin time, 59
Pruritus, 144–145
Psoriasis, 157–158
PT. *See* Prothrombin time
PTT. *See* Partial thromboplastin time
Pulmonary edema, 69
Pulmonary embolism, 62

Quinine poisoning, 228

Radioactive iodine, 147
Raynaud's disease, 176
Raynaud's phenomenon, 166
Refsum's disease
  clinical symptomatology of, 107
  indication for TPE, 89
  treatment of, 107–108
Renal allograft rejection, 193–194
Renal disease
  indication for TPE, 87t
  lupus-associated, 164–165
  TPE for, 178–196
Renal failure, in multiple myeloma,
    186–189
Renal transplantation
  candidate for with cytotoxic
    antibodies, 195–196

focal segmental glomeruloscerlosis after, 192–193
recurrent hemolytic-uremic syndrome with, 126
rejection of, 193–194
Replacement fluids, 28–31
protein-containing, reactions to, 69–70
starch-based solutions as, 35–36
Reticuloendothelial system overloaded, 197
toxic fragments in, 52
Retroperitoneal hemorrhage, 39
Rh disease, 136
Rheumatoid arthritis leukapheresis for, 236
treatment of, 169–170
Rheumatoid vasculitis, severe necrotizing, 170–171
Rheumatologic disorders indication for TPE, 87t
TPE for, 159–176
Rifampin, 38

Scleroderma renal crises of, 167
treatment of, 166–168
Scleroderma antibody (SCL-70), 166
Sensorineural hearing loss, 106–107
Sepsis, 202t
Septic shock, 202t
Septic syndromes, 197
TPE for, 201–203
Sickle cell disease, 238–239
Silver sulfadiazine, 38
Sodium chlorate intoxication, 229
Sodium valproate, 80t
Splenectomy for idiopathic thrombocytopenic purpura, 129
for thrombotic thrombocytopenic purpura, 118
Staphylococcal protein A immunoadsorbant system, 130–131
Staphylococcus aureus infection

protein released from, 45
in temporary vascular catheters, 38
Starch replacement, 35–36
Steroids for idiopathic thrombocytopenic purpura, 129
for lupus-related renal disease, 165
for rapidly progressive glomerulonephritis, 183
for renal failure with multiple myeloma, 187
for vasculitis, 173–174
Stiff-man syndrome indication for TPE, 89
treatment of, 103–104
Streptococcus infection, 38
Streptokinase, 80t
Subclavian catheters, 40
Systemic lupus erythematosus immunoglobulin levels in, 15
treatment of, 159–161

Takayasu's disease, 172
Techniques, 18–52. See also specific techniques
Theophylline poisoning, 229
Therapeutic plasma exchange adverse reactions to, 74
AMA review of efficacy of, 85
anticoagulation in, 26–28
benefits of, 3
centrifugal systems for, 19–20
for chronic inflammatory demyelinating polyneuropathy, 96–97
complications and management of, 53–77
death with, 76–77
for dermatologic disorders, 151–158
with dialysis equipment, 23–25
drug kinetics with, 78
drug removal during, 78–81
fresh frozen plasma in, 32–34
guidelines for prescribing, 5–16
for hematologic disorders, 110–138
in HIV patients, 206–211

Therapeutic plasma exchange
(*continued*)
hollow fiber for, 21f
hypotension during, 75–76
immunoglobulin removal by, 8f
indications for, 86–88t
indications for in ICU, 197–205
indications for in intoxications,
214–232
infection with, 64–66
for metabolic disorders, 139–149
for neurologic disorders, 89–108
prescription for immunoglobulin
removal, 13–16
rational approach to, 10–11
rationale for, 3–4
for renal disease, 178–196
replacement fluids in, 28–31
for rheumatologic disorders, 159–176
serum decline of substance after,
8–10
serum levels of factors after, 59–60
starch replacement for, 35–36
stimulating pathogenic antibody
production, 15–16
technique for, 18–52
traditional method of, 18
vascular access for, 36–41
viral transmission during, 65–66
Thermofiltration, 50
Thrombocytopenia, 60
filter-related, 74
in pregnancy, 122–123
Thrombocytopenic purpura
idiopathic
causes of, 129
in pregnancy, 122–123
treatment of, 129–131
immune, 209
thrombotic
fresh frozen plasma for, 32
in HIV patients, 209–210
lupus-associated, 160
pathogenesis of, 118–119
in pregnancy, 122–123
treatment of, 119–121

Thrombomodulin, 118–119
Thrombopheresis, 237–238
Thrombosis, post-treatment, 62
Thyroid storm, 147–148
Thyrotoxicosis, 147–148
Thyroxine
overdose of, 230
removal during TPE, 81
serum half-life of, 147–148
Tissue plasminogen activator
lack of in TTP, 118–119
recombinant type, with vascular
catheters, 38–39
Tobramycin, 80
Tolbutamide, 80t
Toxic epidermal necrolysis
drug-induced, 155
treatment of, 155–156
TPE. *See* Therapeutic plasma exchange
Transmembrane pressure (TMP),
24–25
Trichloroethylene intoxication, 231
Tricyclic antidepressant overdose,
230–231
Triglycerides, elevated levels of, 144

Ultrafiltration mode, isolated, 23
Ultraviolet light, 145
Urokinase, 38
Uroporphyrin reduction, 156–157
Uroporphyrinogen decarboxylase, 156
Ursodeoxycholic acid, 145
Urticaria, 53

Vanadate intoxication, 231
Vancomycin, 81
Vascular access
antecubital veins, 36–37
permanent arteriovenous, 41
temporary vascular catheters in,
37–40
for TPE with dialysis equipment,
25
Vascular collapse, 205
Vasculitis
rheumatoid, 170–171

systemic, 178
  categories of, 172
  clinical expression of, 172–173
  treatment of, 173–174
Verapamil intoxication, 231
Vinca alkaloids, 129
Vincristine overdose, 231
Viral transmission
  with albumin preparations, 31
  with fresh frozen plasma, 33–34

risk of, 65–66
Vitamin B_{12} removal, 73, 79t
Vitamins, removal of, 73
von Willebrand factor, 118

Waldenström's macroglobulinemia
  2-chlorodeoxyadenosine for, 113
  treatment of, 98–99
Warfarin, 80t
Warm agglutinins, 134–135